INTERNATIONAL
PRIMARY
CARE
COMPUTING

INTERNATIONAL PRIMARY CARE COMPUTING

Proceedings of the IMIA Workshop on
Primary Care Computing
Brighton, United Kingdom, 5 april, 1990

Edited by

G.M. HAYES
Lowesmoore Medical Centre
Lowesmoore, Worcester, U.K.

N. ROBINSON
The Jersey Practice
Hounslow, Middlesex, U.K.

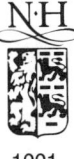

1991

NORTH-HOLLAND
AMSTERDAM • NEW YORK • OXFORD • TOKYO

ELSEVIER SCIENCE PUBLISHERS B.V.
Sara Burgerhartstraat 25
P.O. Box 211, 1000 AE Amsterdam, The Netherlands

Distributors for the United States and Canada:
ELSEVIER SCIENCE PUBLISHING COMPANY INC.
655 Avenue of the Americas
New York, N.Y. 10010, U.S.A.

ISBN: 0 444 89147 1

Printed in the Netherlands

INTRODUCTION

The desire to hold an international meeting in Primary Care Computing had been in our minds for many years. We felt that primary care, or Ambulatory care as it is sometimes called, is a rapidly developing area of information technology. However the needs of workers in primary care are often very different from the needs of workers in hospital or secondary care. Most of the effort and investment in health computing is made in secondary care. As a result primary care is often poorly understood and ignored by many in the IT field.

The concept of 'primary care' differs in different parts of the World. In the developed countries most of the workers in primary care are highly trained doctors and paramedical staff who cope with the majority of patient contacts with health services.
In the developing countries primary care also provides for the majority of episodes of health care but the care is delivered by poorly trained workers who do not have advanced skills. These 'barefoot' doctors are often working many hundreds of miles from the nearest qualified doctor or hospital. They will function with only a limited repertoire of equipment and medications.

These two extremes of primary care workers both need comprehensive computer support. At first sight their needs may appear very different but on closer examination the needs are virtually identical in terms of applications. The differences are in the types of information to be provided and the amount of resources available to fund the applications.

Thus the major aspects of computing which apply to primary care world wide are:

The need to have effective recording of patients on going medical histories.

Medical records in primary care have always been hindered by the wide variety of types of care delivered by a wide variety of carers. Doctors, nurses, welfare workers, physiotherapists, paramedical staff, all tend to be involved in the care of people in their home environments. It may be that the patient visits a doctor in his office in Europe or attends a clinic in South America or is visited by a barefoot doctor in Mongolia. The same need exists to be able to record the patients health events in such a way that:

1. There are checks that protocols for investigation and management of disease are being followed.

2. Children must receive the routine vaccinations advised. Adults with hypertension need their blood pressure monitoring. Treatment given for malaria needs to be assessed.

3. All the medical workers involved in that patients care are aware of each others actions.

Primary Care is provided by workers who are either isolated from other health workers or at the most part of small teams. This isolation can lead to misunderstandings about individual patients.

4. Information is acquired for audit to improve the standards of care.

The very isolation of primary care workers encourages decreasing use of skills and up to date knowledge. Workers in secondary care tend to stimulate each other.

5. Information is collected to improve and develop our understanding of disease.

Most of our present understanding of disease comes from studies which have taken place on patients who have been pre-selected by attendance at hospital. Disease as it occurs in the patient's own environment is much less well understood. Information systems give us the opportunity to develop our understanding of disease.

The need to have information available to a health worker.
No one person can carry all medical knowledge in their head. It may be that a Western doctor needs to be able to look up details of a complicated drug and the worker in the developing country needs to check on the meaning of a set of symptoms. The information may differ but the application of the technology is the same.

The need to have computerised checks on projected actions.
Computers do not sleep, become irritable or forget. Their ability to prompt information to a health worker can vastly improve the quality of care delivered. A prompt to warn that two drugs may interact can save both morbidity and expense. A prompt that a patient is not up to date with their immunisations can save a life.

The need to be able to communicate with other health workers.
I have already mentioned the need to communicate within the primary care sector as one of the functions of a computerised medical record. Workers in primary care will also need to be able to consult with hospital staff. It may be to inform those staff about a patient who is about to enter hospital. There will also be the need to consult on the significance of signs symptoms and investigations. The need to be able to transmit images as well as text may seem only relevant to advanced Western medicine. However the barefoot doctor can function much more effectively if they can transmit such information as ECGs (EKGs) to a distant hospital for analysis.

Thus the need for information technology is universal in primary care. It is also different form the sort of support required in hospitals. Large administrative databases are irrelevant. Complex means of handling complicated cases are not needed. Intensive care has little place in the primary care environment!

Primary Care workers need to get together and shout for their particular needs.

British Primary/Ambulatory Care has always been an active discipline. It is not surprising that computer system amongst British general practitioners are probably more advanced than anywhere else in the world.

The British Computer Society is the professional computing body for the UK and has various medical Specialist Groups. These groups come together under the umbrella of the Health Informatics Specialist Group(HISG) which provide the British representative to the International Medical Informatics Association (IMIA).

Each year the HISG holds a major computing exhibition called Health Computing (HC). When the members of the primary health care specialist Group(PHCSG) decided that they wanted to hold an international conference the logical step was to suggest to HISG that this international meeting should form part of the health Computing Conference. This was agreed in principle in 1988.

Several members of the PHCSG attended the MEDINFO 89 conference in Singapore. At MEDINFO 89 we held a workshop on Primary Care. This was attended by 28 workers from around the world.(Table 1.) All of the participants came from developed countries but Dr Mandil from WHO was able to point out many of the differences between the participants view of life and the problems of workers in developing countries.

Definition of Primary Care
The group discussed this at length. Each country had its own definition. There was a major distinction between the developed countries who described primary care as that provide by doctors and attached ancillary medical workers from an office rather that a hospital, and developing Nations who has the view that primary care did not require medical staff but was considered to be any care which could be taken to the patient away form large centres. It was therefore decide that Primary Care includes:

First point of patients contact.

Not an in-patient

No fixed diagnosis/symptoms - fuzzy sets

not necessarily involving a doctor.

The workshop went on to discuss the problems primary care workers had with implementing computer systems. As the attenders were not representative of developing countries the list of problems they produced Table 2.is obviously biased towards the developed countries.

Table 2. What are the problems limiting doctor use of Primary Care Systems?

Need for adequate minimum data sets.

Dislike of keyboards

Disinterest, not willing to see the benefits.

Unwillingness to accept technology by both patients and governments.

Cost implications

Systems not showing significant benefits except in administration

IMIA has a number of Working groups which explore various specialised areas of International Health Computing. Working group 5, under the Chairmanship of Peter Reichertz, had been concerned with Ambulatory care. Following his death the Working Group had been inactive. The workshop in Singapore suggested that there could be a place for a Working group in Primary Care.

This would promote the benefits of primary care systems to patients, professionals and governments. If information about activities and proven benefits are disseminated internationally the results could be used by workers to put pressure on those with influence in their homelands.

Possible functions of Working Group 5

To encourage the development of internationally agreed data transfer standards / coding systems.

To encourage the development of computer systems by disseminating ideas and information about world-wide activities.

To consider difficulties such as the problems of data entry.

TABLE 1 Attendance at the Singapore Workshop in Primary Care Computing.

This table also show the percentage of GPs in each country who use a computer as perceived by the workshop attenders.

	GP	Other Doctor	Computer Professional	Computerised % Practices
Eng & Wales	2		1	45
Scotland	1			42
USA	1	1		35
Japan	1	1		30-50
FR Germany			1	10
NZ	1		1	20
Australia	2			20-30
S. Africa	1		1	50
Sweden	1			>5
Israel	2			2
Canada	1			35
Norway		1		10
Finland			1	10-20
Holland			1	10-15
WHO			1	
	===	===	===	
total	13	3	7	

It is not surprising that, with exception of the UK, the countries which required the doctor to bill the patient had the highest proportion of GPs who are computerised. The UK has a high take up of clinical computers partly because of funding initiatives and partly because the UK system of lists of registered patients ensures that British GPs provide 90% of health care contacts. This on-going care encourages the use of clinical systems.

It had already been decided by the British that the Health Computing Conference scheduled for April 1990 would be a meeting concerned with International Primary Care Computing. After the Singapore Workshop a proposal was put to the IMIA board that an IMIA Working Conference should be arranged for the day after the HC90 conference. Part of the remit for this conference would be to consider the possibility of re-constituting Working Group 5 if the need was substantiated.

The total attendance at HC90 was 1200 delegates. A few of these delegate were invited to stay for the IMIA Working conference. The format of this conference was a series of workshops. See Table 3.

For each Workshop there was appointed a Chairman, and a rapporteur. Also, one distinguished guest presented a paper to open the session. Following this another guest acted as discussant to provide a controversial view. The session was then thrown open to the floor.

The Chairman was responsible for co-ordinating the report on the session with the rapporteur. As a result these proceeding consist of one or all of the following:

A Chairman's report.

A paper from the first speaker

A paper from the Discussant

A report from the rapporteur.

In some case these reports or papers have not been submitted so there are gaps in some of the session documents. At the end of each session the delegates came together for a plenary session which is reported in brief at the end of the main proceedings.

It was apparent to many of us that there is very little organised information on primary care computing. As a result a student at the University of Manchester Science and Technology,(UMIST) carried out a project to prepare a bibliography of our subject. We feel that it can form the basis of a more organised future. It is in two parts. It begins with an author index arranged by subject. There is then a description of each entry in more detail.

Finally at the end of this book we include the letter sent to IMIA from the Working Conference. We hope that you find this book stimulating and rewarding.

Glyn Hayes	Nicholas Robinson.
Chairman	Secretary PHCSG
3 Beech Avenue North	The Jersey Practice
Worcester	484 Great West Rd
WR3 8PX	Hounslow, Middlesex
UK	UK
Tel + 44 905-54705	+ 44 81 577 5431
Fax + 44 905-56817	+ 44 81 569 6251

TABLE OF CONTENTS

Session Titles and Main Participants in IMIA Working Conference on Primary Care Computing

5th April 1990

Session One , Interfacing Doctors to Computer Systems.

- **Chairman** :Dr M.Fitter, MRC/ESRC Applied Psychology Unit Dept. of Psychology University of Sheffield Sheffield S10 2TN UK
- **Presenter** :Dr A. Rector, Medical Informatics Group Dept. of Computer Science Manchester University Oxford Road Manchester M13 9PL UK

- **Discussant:**Dr M. O'Neil, Imperial Cancer Research Fund 44 Lincolns Inn Fields London WC2A 3PX UK
- **Rapporteur:**Dr Neill Jones, Marsden Road Health Centre Marsden Road South Shields SR6 7PN. UK

Session Two. Decision Support

- **Chairman** :Dr Bob Johnson, Thorns 16c Clough Lane Grasscroft Oldham OL4 3EW UK
- **Presenter** :Dr Rolfe Engelbrecht, GSF-MEDIS Ingoldstadter Landstr 1 8042 Neuherberg Germany
- **Discussant:**Dr A. Glowinski, Imperial Cancer Research Fund 44 Lincolns Inn Fields London WC2A 3PX UK
- **Rapporteur:**Dr Nick Booth, Willow Lodge Hallyards Farm Stocksfield Northumberland NE43 7LR UK

Session Three. Coding and Classification

- **Chairman** :Dr A.Nowlan, Medical Informatics Group Dept. of Computer Science Manchester University Oxford Road Manchester M13 9PL UK
- **Presenter** :Dr R. Weeks, 9 Upper Brighton Road Surbiton Surrey KT6 6LQ UK
- **Discussant:**Dr S. Shepherd, 169 Long Ashton Road Long Ashton Bristol BS18 9JQ UK
- **Rapporteur,** Dr. M Bainbridge , The Surgery Hexton Road Barton Beds.

Session Four, Screening

- **Chairman** :Prof. B. Richards, Dept. of Computer Science UMIST Sackville Street Manchester M60 1QD UK
- **Presenter** :Dr M. Fitter, MRC/ESRC Applied Psychology Unit Dept. of Psychology University of Sheffield Sheffield S10 2TN UK
- **Discussant:**Dr M. Crampton, 34 Amesbury Avenue Sefton New South Wales 2162 Australia
- **Rapporteur:**Mrs A. Daniels, Oxford Community Health Project Oxford RHA Old Road Headington Oxford

Session Five , Medical Audit

- **Chairman** :Mr S. Kay, Medical Informatics Group Dept. of Computer Science Manchester University Oxford Road Manchester M13 9PL UK
- **Presenter** :Dr G. Page, 9 Nightingale Lane Earlsden Coventry CV9 6AY UK
- **Discussant**:Dr M. Lawrence, West Street Surgery 12 West Street Chipping Norton Oxon. OX7 5AA UK
- **Rapporteur**:Dr R. Bowles, Upper Knapps Shire Lane Lyme Regis Dorset DT7 3ET UK

Session Six, Communications

- **Chairman** :Prof. P. Grob, Robens Institute University of Surrey Guildford Surrey UK
- **Presenter** :Dr A. Stokes, 97 Mill Way Mill Hill London NW7 3JL UK
- **Discussant**:Dr D. Markwell, 93 Wantage Road Reading Berks. UK
- **Rapporteur**:Mr H. Ward, Forge Cottage Westbrook Street Blewbury Oxon. OX11 9QB UK

Session Seven, IT for Development

- **Chairman** :Prof. Z. Ibrahim, Institute of Child Health Great Ormond Street London UK
- **Presenter** :Prof. Otto Rienhoff, Institute of Medical Informatics Phillips Universtat FB Humanmedizin und Klinikum Bunsenstrasse 3, D-3550 Marburg West Germany
- **Discussant**:Dr R. Brittain, North Warwickshire Health Authority Heath End Road Nuneaton UK
- **Discussant**:Mr R. Fawdry, Milton Keynes Hospital Milton Keynes Bucks. UK
- **Rapporteur**:Ms Grizelda Moules, Raspberry Cottage 87 Corsham Road Whitley Melksham Wilts. SN12 8QF UK

Session Eight, Demography & IT

- **Chairman** :Dr G. Dove, North End Medical Centre 211 North End Road London W14 9WT UK
- **Presenter** :Prof. B.Jarman, Lisson Grove Health Centre Gateforth Street London NW8 8EG UK
- **Discussant**:Dr R. Turner, Hull Health Authority Victoria House Park Street Hull HU2 8TD UK
- **Rapporteur**:Dr B. Higginson, 45 Wellington Sq. Hastings, East Sussex, TN34 1PN UK

Session Nine, Medical Records

- **Chairman** :Dr Alan Rector, Medical Informatics Group Dept. of Computer Science Manchester University Oxford Road Manchester M13 9PL UK

- **Presenter** :Mrs Sheila Warshawsky, Faculty of Health Sciences Ben Gurion University of the Negev Beersheva Israel.
- **Discussant**:Dr Stuart Foote, Heretaunga Medical Centre 306 West Lyndon Road Hastings New Zealand
- **Rapporteur**:Dr John Williams, 1 Woodruff Avenue Guildford Surrey GU1 1XS UK

Session Ten, Security & Data Protection
- **Chairman** :Dr Rory O'Moore, Dept. of Biochemistry St.James' Hospital James Street PO Box 580 Dublin 8
- **Presenter** :Dr Barry Barber, NHS Information Management Centre 19 Calthorpe Road Edgbaston Birmingham B15 1RP UK
- **Discussant**:Dr Nigel Harding, 82 Lime Walk, Oxford OX3 7AY UK
- **Rapporteur**:Dr Glyn Hayes, 3 Beech Avenue North, Worcester WR3 8PX, UK

Session Eleven, Education about and through IT
- **Chairman** :Prof. S. Khaihara, University Hospital Computer Center, Tokyo 113 Japan
- **Presenter** :Mrs E. Pluyter-Wenting, Bazis Foundation PO Box 901 2300 AX Leiden The Netherlands
- **Discussant**:Mr Alan Mcwilliams, Dept. of General Practice New Medical School Ashton Street Liverpool UK
- **Rapporteur**:Dr I. Goodman, Northwood Medical Centre, Northwood, Middlesex, UK

Session Twelve, Research Use of Routine Data
- **Chairman** :Dr Neill Jones, Marsden Road Health Centre, South Shields, SR6 7PN UK.
- **Presenter** :Dr Ian Black, AAH Meditel Rigby Hall Rigby Lane Bromsgrove Worcs. B60 2EW UK
- **Discussant**:Dr Gillian Hall, VAMP Health Ltd. The Bread Factory 1a Broughton Street London SW8 3QT UK

Other participants included:
Mr Bud Abbott, 55 Fore St. Hartland. Bideford Devon. EX39 4BD UK
Mr M Rigby, NHS IMC 19 Calthorpe Rd, Birmingham UK
Dr Gunnar Wellander, Hornsg. 20 Box 70487 10726 Stockholm, Sweden
Mr Peter Kjaer, Einarsvej 18, Dk 2800, Lynaby, Copenhagen Denmark
Dr D Robson, Greenwich District Hospital, London SE10 9HE UK
Dr Allon Zuker, Roshtov Software Ltd.,31 Smilanski St. Beersheva 84213 Israel
Dr J Van Damme, University of Leuven, 3000 Leuven Belgium.

International Primary Care Computing
G.M. Hayes and N. Robinson (Editors)
Elsevier Science Publishers B.V. (North-Holland)
© IMIA, 1991

1   INTERFACING DOCTORS TO COMPUTER SYSTEMS

1.1   Intelligent Clinical Data Entry for General Practice: The PEN Project

B. Horan, A. Nowlan, A. Wilson, E. Sneath, A. Rector, C. Goble, T. Howkins, S. Kay

Medical Informatics Group, University of Manchester, MANCHESTER, M13 9PL, United Kingdom

Abstract

The PEN1 and PAD2 projects [1] are employing user-centered design techniques to develop a prototype computerised information environment for general practitioners. The goal is to design the desktop workstation which will be used by doctors in the next decade. The model centres on an "Intelligent Medical Record" which will ultimately replace most of the existing paper records. The system will provide a single integrated environment within which other communication and decision-support systems used by doctors in the consulting room can be accommodated. This paper reports on the data entry techniques developed within the PEN and PAD projects to date, and discusses their success. We conclude by describing the unexpected user acceptance for a form-filling dialogue, and the extent to which that metaphor was extended.

Introduction

Computer-based clinical systems need to hold comprehensive, detailed, and highly structured patient information before they can be truly useful for individual and practice-wide patient care. However, one of the major concerns of doctors wishing or being required to extend their use of computer systems for clinical care, is the time and effort required for such comprehensive data entry, particularly during the consultation. Working under severe time and resource limitations, doctors are naturally unwilling or unable to divert their attention from the primary task of direct patient care [2].

At the heart of the PEN project is the belief that GPs will only be prepared to enter detailed information if they are provided with quick and easy-to-use techniques for doing so. Ideally, a doctor should be able to deal with the common types of consultation at least as quickly as with conventional records.

General User Interface Requirements

A serious criticism of many computer-based clinical systems is their tendency to impose a rigid, hierarchical, and sequential ordering on the tasks a doctor may wish to perform during a consultation. This need for flexibility resulted in a minimum set of requirements:

- the system should not impose a fixed sequence upon the many tasks which the user may wish to perform during a consultation.

- the system should allow the user to deal with several tasks in parallel and to switch easily between them.

- the system should not compel the user to enter information which he or she does not wish to enter.

These requirements have been met by the adoption of a window-based environment, which allows multiple tasks to be dealt with in multiple windows. Consequently, user interaction is non-modal - the user does not need to complete one task before beginning another. The use of forms, graphics, and "point & select" techniques allows the user to move rapidly between tasks, minimises keyboard use, and causes less intrusion in the doctor-patient relationship.

Clinical Data Entry

The "consultation" is a generic term covering many types of and reasons for a patient contact. This heterogeneity implies that a single approach to clinical data entry is inappropriate. To explore this further we employed a simple taxonomy of consultations:

1. New, straightforward, common problem, e.g. urinary tract infection

2. New, complex (potentially serious) problem, e.g. chest pain

3. Follow-up of an acute episode, e.g. one week review of treated bronchitis

4. Follow-up for management of a chronic or recurrent complaint, e.g. diabetic check-up

Our research on data entry has so far concentrated on the new presentations of problems described in 1 and 2 above. Entering information on a new complaint can be broadly divided into two steps: (i) entering the main topic or problem (e.g. cough), and (ii) adding further detail, if required (e.g. for 3 days, with no sputum).

(i)Entering the Main Topic (Telling the System what I want to talk about)
The problem of navigating large medical classifications, or their equivalent, is a notoriously difficult one. Traditional approaches adopt a mixture of using alphabetical or keyword search, and browsing a hierarchical classification by successive refinement. The underlying model of the PEN and PAD architecture supports the development of novel tools to tackle this problem. We describe two methods: simple data entry for common consultations, and a complex method for the more general case.

Common Consultations - the "Quickies"
A large percentage of General Practice consultations are accounted for by a relatively small number of complaints, which is reflected in the users' requests for a short-list of the most

common complaints. The contents of the short-list should not be fixed, and must be tailorable to the individual doctor. The current implementation is via a simple menu, called the "Quickies Menu", available from a menu bar. It contains a heterogenous list of topics, from which it is possible to select more than one item at a time. Having done so, the user may add the statements to the record or proceed to add more detail using the form filling dialogue described below.

A General Method - the Graphical Entry Tool
During workshops the doctors frequently requested diagrams to assist with data entry. They outlined at least three uses for such a diagrammatic tool.

1. As a means of locating the site of a specific symptom, e.g. placing a rash on the arm
2. As a means of selecting a symptom by selecting its location, e.g. selecting the ear to obtain earache
3. As a decision support tool, e.g. tell me what is wrong with the ear

The Graphical Entry Tool (GET) originated within the design team and was based on the second of these ideas (see figure 1). It was conceived as a mechanism for searching through medical concepts such as diagnoses and symptoms using diagrams, and has no analogue within paper records. The GET has stimulated a large variety of responses and opinions over its use and interpretation. In functional terms the GET is purely a means of browsing a bi-axial model for categorising symptoms and diagnoses. Its axes are the physiological system and topographical area of the body and the medical model is more closely related to the SNOMED [3] approach to medical descriptions than to a traditional classification (although it uses much tighter definitions and more consistent semantics).

The GETs interface style is similar to that used in the Stanford Anatomy Project [4], but its functionality is quite different. It can be used to identify the site and, if appropriate, the laterality of the problem. Movement along either axis is independent of the other, overcoming some of the restrictions imposed by uni-axial classification browsers. By using familiar metaphors, the GET attempts to help doctors focus quickly on the context. The current implementation allows the user to specify a major physiological system from the row of endomorphs, and an area of the body by either clicking on that area or selecting it from the adjacent list. Menus of pertinent diseases or symptoms are then generated by the GET using its knowledge base and the specified context (e.g. the combination of the musculoskeletal system and the elbow produces musculoskeletal diseases and symptoms of the elbow, such as osteoarthrosis, tennis elbow etc).

The doctors' response to the GET was enthusiastic, although many viewed it as a decision support tool - a purpose for which it was not intended. Work is continuing to develop both the conceptual model and its implementation.

(ii) Adding Further Detail   (The Form-Filling Approach)
The form-filling mechanism (see figure 2) was created originally to facilitate the speedy entry of details pertaining to a new problem. The provisional model and the content for a few conditions were developed in user workshops through the use of patient scenarios and protocols. These were then modified and translated into the form-based data entry.

The forms are divided into areas covering the description of the particular symptom, sets of related symptoms, signs etc. The user interacts with the form by using the mouse to press buttons, access menus and move sliders. It would be impossible to define explicitly suitable protocols for all encounters in general practice, and a major development was the linking of the forms to a knowledge-based mechanism for generating their content. It is not intended that this should be the only method by which a form is created; however it does allow the system to create sensible forms for most situations. The functionality of the forms has been extended recently so that they are also able to indicate the state of any pertinent, previously entered data.

In the future, the content of the forms will be tailorable by the user. The current knowledge-base is very small (less than 1,000 nodes and links) and thus the medical content of the forms is limited.

Despite their earlier scepticism, the doctors were amenable to data entry based on pre-defined choices. The choice of interaction style had removed much of the rigidity associated with traditional computerised data entry forms. The majority of the early forms were quite detailed, but the variation in response to this level of detail depended chiefly on the perceived significance of the symptom, rather than on the differences between doctors.

For example, the level of detail for chest pain was felt to be appropriate whereas earache was considered too detailed. Although the user was under no obligation to attend to any one item, it was sometimes difficult to identify the items of key interest. This is the area where "layering" of detail will be vital in making systems quick for common situations. Nonetheless, most users were impressed with the level of detail that could be entered through this mechanism. Figure 3 shows the result of accepting the content of the form in figure 2.

Discussion

Great importance was attached to the forms' potential for cueing and prompting the doctor, and thus reducing mistakes and omissions. However, concern was also expressed over the potential rail-roading effect of such a technique, which could make doctors less likely to consider other possibilities or relevant factors. Overall, the benefits were considered likely to outweigh this potential drawback. It is clear that doctors can vary widely in what they wish to record or consider during a consultation. Many of their opinions are highly idiosyncratic, but no less valid for being so. It is thus important that the content of the data entry mechanism, together with most of the rest of the system, be tailorable by the individual doctor or practice, and that the system-generated forms can be seen as the basis for adaptation.

Although at present the time taken for the system to produce the forms is not excessive, further evaluation must be undertaken to discover whether the use of a larger knowledge base will cause an unacceptable delay. To date, research has focussed on data entry for new problems. Plans for future development include the integration of data display and entry so that all elements support both of these (e.g. entering a new Blood Pressure on a display of previous Blood Pressures) and the utilisation of summarisation and problem lists to initiate data-entry. As well as introducing user controllable tailorability of the interface and medical content, it is also intended to provide support for the annotation of any item with free-text. Research on both the current and new data entry techniques, including the GET, will also be developed and extended. Data entry on long standing problems that is both quick and contextually appropriate, depends on successful techniques for the summarisation and manipulation of complex histories. These form a major part of the PAD project and are the subject of current research. The success of data entry techniques developed for use in demanding environments such as the General Practice consulting room can only be truly measured when used in situ. However, our experiences lead to the belief that a forms-based data entry mechanism can increase the acceptability of computer-based clinical information systems in the consulting room.

References

1. Kay B, Horan B et al, A Consulting Room System with Added Value, paper submitted to Medical Informatics Europe '90.

2. Rector A L, Helping with a Humanly Impossible Task: Integrating Knowledge Base Systems into Clinical Care. In J Hanmu & L Seppo (Eds), Proceedings of the Second Scandinavian Conference on Artificial Intelligence, Tampere, Finland, pp 560-572.

3. College of American Pathologists. Systematized nomenclature of medicine.(first edition). Skokie, Illinois, USA: College of American Pathologists, 1977

4. Chase RA, Freedman SJ. Electric Cadaver: A dynamic book of human structure and function. Advanced Media Research Group, Division of Human Anatomy, Stanford University School of Medicine, Stanford, 1986.1

Acknowledgements

1.Practitioners Entering Notes, is supported by The Department of Health

2.Practitioners Accessing Data, is supported by the Medical Research Council

International Primary Care Computing
G.M. Hayes and N. Robinson (Editors)
Elsevier Science Publishers B.V. (North-Holland)
© IMIA, 1991

1.2 Interfacing Doctors to Computer Systems: Report

Chairman, Dr Mike Fitter

MRC/ESRC Applied Psychology Unit Dept. of Psychology University of Sheffield
Sheffield S10 2TN, UK

Presenter, Dr Alan Rector

Medical Informatics Group Dept. of Computer Science Manchester University Oxford
Road Manchester M13 9PL, UK

Discussant, Dr Mike O'Neil

Imperial Cancer Research Fund 44 Lincolns Inn Fields London WC2A3PX, UK

Rapporteur, Dr Neill Jones

Marsden Road Health Centre Marsden Road South Shields SR6 7PN. UK.

Chairman's Opening Remarks

There are four questions we need to answer today:

> Why?
> Who?
> When?
> How?

Why Do we Collect Data?
There are two main reasons why data is collected: first for patient care, and second for audit
and epidemiological research.

Who will be Using the Data?
Many different types of doctor and many different specialists. Each will have different
needs and different styles of use. All other primary care workers may need and want to
record patient information and their different needs and styles need to be catered for.

When will the Information be Recorded and Retrieved?
The information can be accessed before, during, or after the patient contact. Generally it is considered better if the information can be recorded at the time of contact. In this way it is likely to be more complete and accurate.

How to Produce the Interface?
This is the real challenge to software engineers - to design a structure to cope with all these needs.

The Interface Between the Computer and the User

The Interface
The interface must be concerned with usability. This will be judged by the user.

The Environment
The environment is concerned with the usefulness of the system interface. The usability to be judged again by the user.

The Benefits
The overall benefits will be judged by society, by colleagues as well as the users.

The Users of the System

Up to the present the users of computers in medicine have fallen into two camps: the expert and the novice. In the future all shades of user, frequent and infrequent, will need to be accommodated.

What Does the Ideal System have to Do?

Be Quick
How fast is the machine; how many mistakes do the users make; is it painful to use. The system must not overload the user and it must avoid increasing the work done.

Be Flexible
Current database expert systems need to do many different things concurrently. They should not force the user in a specific direction, so should be flexible in the use of any mode at any time. It is important to look at the downside when developing any system.

The Goal of any Interface

The interface is a good system when some other aspect of the system is noticed and the interface is invisible. Or if the system is only noticed by its absence when, for example, the computer is not working.

There are many different user requirements and there needs to be many different levels of user configurability.

Discussion

The session continued with a very lively debate. The following is a summary of the main points.

The Interface Development

The learning curve for a new interface is 1 to 3 weeks. Despite this it is important to have compatibility across systems so when users move they can use the new system easily. This can be a long-term migration to a new system or the temporary change while in a different work place.

It is important to remember that doctors are not good designers and that doctors are not the only users. The designers need to develop systems that can be used by all users now and as their experience grows and their needs change because system requirement by the user changes with time and use.

The Data

A very flexible system is not compatible with standardisation of recording. The underlying structure needs to be integral but the view the interface places on that data needs to be different to each of the different type of user. There needs to be some formal structure imposed on the data for all users and there needs to be a structure that a group of users can impose on their own data so that they can formalise the way they use that information and hence improve the value of their data. However a user interface that is completely different across multiple sites causes many problems to users of more than one system at once.

Transferring data between systems permanently and temporarily has several problems at present. Accessibility of data is the most important reason for the recording of that information and any system that is unable to output the data held in the form the user requires has failed. Communication between systems requires data extraction so there needs to be a minimum data report format so that comparative data can be produced across the system and transferred easily between systems.

The adoption of the Read codes requires a description of the codes; their meaning; the correct and incorrect uses they can be put to; and how best to implement their use.

Further work needs to be done on the recording of data, the qualifiers that systems place on that data, and how this data can be transferred.

The Consultation and Using the Interface

The computer interaction and the effect on the consultation needs to be addressed, especially the long term changes to consultation techniques. The education of students and trainees about computers and information technology is very necessary, as is the continuing education of all users. There is no current co-ordination of IT medical education. Some data needs to be collected for others and this needs to be explained to the users to get their full co-operation.

Presentation

Mike O'Neil is a designer on the Oxford System of Medicine project, a generalised decision support capability for primary care physicians using principles from artificial intelligence.

Mike described a way of considering the interface in which stress was laid on the importance of providing support for the tasks carried out in the consultation, and of integrating use of the computer into the processes of the consultation. The critical considerations were considered to be not which devices (mouse, keyboard), nor which screen layout should be used, but which consultation tasks should be supported and what kind of knowledge representation would be needed to underpin the data entry, reporting and decision support tasks that a computer system might carry out.

A starting point was Moran's Command Language Grammar, one method for analysing and designing a user interface. His definition of an interface is "The system as the user sees it" and four levels of analysis are considered. These, listed below, analyse an interface at increasing levels of detail.

Conceptual Component

> - Task level (a description of the tasks to be handled by the system)

> - Semantic level (a description of the objects and terms that appear at the interf

Communication Component

> - Syntactic level (e.g. system commands, arguments, and contexts)

> - Interaction level (e.g. sequence of key presses required)

Physical Component

> - Spatial layout (e.g. windows)

- Device level (e.g. mouse, keyboard, screen)

In keeping with this approach, Mike proposed an analysis of the tasks of the consultation in primary care from the viewpoint of the practitioner who is the potential system user. These consisted of:

Communication tasks
- Reassuring the patient
- Extracting information, ideas and perceptions from the patient
- Involving the patient

Medical tasks
- Reactive, preventative
- Diagnosis, investigation, treatment, prescribing, screening, referral

Office tasks
- Recording (symptoms, diagnoses, treatments, views)
- Reading (notes)
- Requesting (lab results, physiotherapy)
- Reporting (assurance reports, letters)

Information Seeking tasks
- Drug doses, addresses, regulations
- Symptom prompts, management suggestions

Learning tasks
- From hospital letters, formularies - e.g. some drug doses

Finally, a set of principles that a successful user interface will need to adhere to was described, based upon analyses and critical evaluations of the OSM's interface.

Maximise flexibility
Allow the user "to do anything at any time", not constraining him with a particular task sequence as consultation mapping has shown that no perfect task sequence exists for all consultations.

Provide Support in both Executive and Decision-making Tasks
Though providing decision support is a laudable aim, direct and perceivable benefits in executive tasks (e.g. automatic generation of letters, assurance reports) are required to counterbalance the demands of extra data entry.

Reduce Cognitive Overload
The task analysis demonstrates the complexity of a GP's job, and requiring him to perform yet more complex tasks (looking for a command hidden in a menu, on another screen; formulating a medical query in a neo-Boolean language) will worsen matters. Report models should therefore reflect the structure of the consultation.

Maximise Configurability
General practitioners vary in their experience, skills and practice and a single user interface might not be expected to cope ideally with everyone's requirements.

In the discussion following Mike's talk, the following points were made:

1. Configurability has the potential (though not necessary) drawback of not permitting transfer of experience in the best layouts, etc.

2. There was general agreement that the appropriate level of analysis for a user interface was at the level of task description. But the task list was not felt to be complete (for the consultation). In particular it was felt that social tasks had been omitted.

3. The user interface can be designed to be:
- patient lead
- task lead
- outcome lead
- income lead
- or health promotion lead

4. Assessments of interfaces will have to be made, the criteria for which will be the use it has been for the patient and not the doctor.

5. How can the suppliers be controlled, and what mechanism is needed to achieve this?

6. Concentration is needed on what is possible at present, and what may evolve, so that best use is made of current possibilities. Current systems should be improved with our current knowledge rather than create new systems.

7. Migration of information is essential and urgent work on this is needed.

8. Training for all users and potential users needs to be improved. This needs to be coordinated, as current training and education is often seen as poor.

9. Data recording at some levels must be uniform, and this may need to be proscribed by the Government, or some body.

10. The user needs to have ready access to all the data that they have recorded.

Main Conclusions

It is considered better if the information can be recorded at the time of contact.

Many different users need to use the interface.

The interface must be concerned with usability.

The overall benefits will be judged by society.

The system must not overload the user.

The interface should not force the user in a specific direction.

It is important to have some compatibility across systems as configurability has the potential (though not necessary) drawback of not permitting transfer of experience in the best layouts, etc.

The view of recorded data will need to be presented in many different ways to many different users.

Any system that is unable to output the data held in the form the user requires has failed.

Further work needs to be done on advice on how to record data in standard ways.

The long term effect of computers on the consultation needs to be addressed.

The aim is knowledge representation.

The interface should allow the user to define his own pattern of work without constraint.

Training for all users needs to be improved.

International Primary Care Computing
G.M. Hayes and N. Robinson (Editors)
Elsevier Science Publishers B.V. (North-Holland)
© IMIA, 1991

2 DECISION SUPPORT SYSTEMS

Chairman, Bob Johnson

Vice-Chairman, Primary Health Care Specialist Group, British Computer Society

Speaker, Rolf Engelbrecht

GSF-MEDIS Munich

Discussant, Andrezj Glowinski

Imperial Cancer Research Fund 44 Lincolns Inn Fields London WC2A 3PX

Rapporteur: Dr Nick Booth, Willow Lodge Hallyards Farm Stocksfield
Northumberland NE43 7LR

Chairman's Introduction

In General Practice in the UK, 370 million prescriptions are written each year, representing a cost to the nation of approximately £2 billion. This involves about 400,000,000 clinical decisions, relating to around 150 million patient encounters each year, quite apart from the expense of hospital referrals and investigations.

Presentation

Dr Engelbrecht outlined the primary areas to be addressed in the discussion:

1 Quality of Care
2 Cost of Care
3 The Working Environment
4 The Doctor - Patient relationship
5 Ethical and Legal considerations

He outlined his view of the status quo, and presented information obtained from questionnaires and interviews from professionals involved in decision support systems. He has found that most systems are still in a development stage, and few are in routine daily use. Furthermore, most are only used in the institutions in which they have been developed, and few are used outside of that sphere.

It seems that the four main areas of use are

1 Diagnosis

2 Treatment

3 Triage

4 Evaluation

Although most existing operational systems are used in diagnosis, there is a trend of increasing interest in development of treatment systems. He feels that the main future developments will be in therapeutic decision support.

The integration of these systems is an important objective (i.e. with communications and patient records).

Patient centred questionnaires have shown a positive consumer reaction to expert systems, with over 96% approving the use of computer support in the management of insulin dependent diabetics in his own research.

It is to be hoped that as these systems develop, they may be especially useful in areas with low provision of health care. Also there may be an opportunity to increase the proportion of out-patient care in comparison to in-patient care.

In conclusion Dr Engelbrecht emphasised the importance of careful evaluation of new systems before their use was to be relied upon in actual patient care. There will need to be VERIFICATION, VALIDATION, and ASSESSMENT, and a "certificate of integrity" would be needed.

The aim of those involved in future development could be summarised by the tasks mentioned in the proposals at the beginning of the session. The German group is working toward a goal of having a working interface of clinicians and informatics experts by the year 2000.

Discussant Andreij Glowinski -

Knowledge based systems (KBS) have become more mature over the last 20 years, having begun as laboratory based systems, but now finding their way more and more into clinical areas. We need now to face up to the following problems:

1 What is the role of a decision support system? What is the need and what is the effect?

2 How will the support be used to enable 'better decisions'?

3 What will be the degree of integration of these systems?

4 What are the principles of the application of these systems?

5 What are the appropriate evaluation methods before generalised use? (Drug evaluation may be a useful analogy).

Questions posed:

- Does the system address a real clinical problem?
- Which decisions need decision support technology?
- Where does uncertainty arise?
- Where are suboptimal choices being made?
- When are mistakes made?
- Which aspects of a particular health care system impinge upon the role of decision support systems?
- What will be the effects on individual patient care?
- What are the effects on the organisation and delivery of services?

Assumptions

Whereas it may be assumed that decision support may optimise care there may well be a concomitant increase in the cost of care, because of an increased demand on services. Appropriate decisions are not now always being made - we may 'uncover pathology'.

A three dimensional graph was presented which compared integration of all types of support both with integration with other systems and across the domain.

Discussion

Dr Johnson posed the problem of patients inadvertently being placed in the wrong specialist ward with subsequent suboptimal care as their carers are not tuned into the correct pathology, e.g. the patient with dyspeptic type pain on a surgical ward who is in fact suffering from cardiac pain. Could a background system patrol clinical parameters on the clinical system and alert clinicians to alternative possible diagnoses which they have failed to consider?

He reiterated the problem of budgetary pressures encouraging the substitution of out-patient for in-patient care.

Peter Kjaer - As a GP Dr Kjaer felt that too many KBS seemed to focus down on clinical problems rather than take the wider view (? hypothetico-deductive reasoning vs inductive reasoning).

Dr D Robson felt that the three most needed areas of support will be in:

a) Therapy KBS
b) Diagnostic support

c) Pattern of care evaluation (case mix data handling)

Andreij Glowinski emphasised the difference between KBS and Expert systems. The latter ultimately may provide valid second opinions, whereas the former merely prompts useful information, e.g. drug dosage or side effects.
Rolf Engelbrecht: Surely the KBS should work as a background tool only.

David Markwell: He foresees the prime need of an Expert System (EXPS) in giving a confirmatory indication of the patient's 3D position in the breadth of health care. We should allow the clinician to concentrate on the detail of his specialty.

Allon Zuker: In narrow decision support systems one needs to know the diagnosis prior to 'fine tuning'. The problem of developing isolated systems remains. They must be integrated with the main clinical record. When this is achieved, one can then contemplate meaningful prompting from the system, e.g. 'Have you checked the lymph nodes?' This will lead to background monitoring with prompting.

David Markwell: Software techniques are no longer the problem in decision support. However an integrated knowledge base does not exist in a usable form (by these techniques).

Alan Rector: Described his view of the range of forms of support

Monitoring -	Are you missing a killer?
Cueing -	Do what you said you'd do!
Information -	Presents the knowledge you need.
Advice -	Specific or open
Analysis -	Enhancement of available data by improved presentation.

Casebook Reasoning - Look for other patients like this one.

Peter Kjaer: We need to see blood hound programs which look at the clinical data overnight and present cues, or prompts, where appropriate, but otherwise are unobtrusive.

David Robson: There is a risk of overfunding an underevaluated field where costs may be enormous.

Roger Britain: Should we proceed without knowing more clearly where we are going? There seems to be insufficient theoretical or academic thinking addressing the purpose of AI/EXPS. There are no paper analogues for what is going on in Decision Support.

Alan Rector: Since things do go wrong, we will benefit from better provision of information which may help reduce the likelihood of error. We must target those areas where mistakes may lead to serious problems.

Such areas include those where protocols don't get followed, or drug interactions and adverse reactions are missed or under reported.

David Markwell: We need four levels of data:

> Textual Knowledge
> Knowledge network
> Casebook data
> Individual patient data

Mike O'Neil: Text based retrieval may be implemented easily as a first step (e.g. protocols).

Alan Rector: High pay off areas could be addressed first, e.g. cueing, information handling - these are easy to implement. But don't use a computer if a notice in casualty is enough, e.g. "ABDO PAIN - DO AN AMYLASE ! "

Plenary Session

Chairman's closing remarks

We have heard two presentations, the first of which has emphasised the need to VERIFY, VALIDATE and ASSESS decision support systems prior to acceptance as a working tool in clinical practice, and the second of which has urged the integration of KBS into healthcare computer systems.

We have had a wide ranging discussion. Examples of the problems considered: the missed perceptions of a clinician cannot be assimilated by a KBS even though it is available to the clinician. The second is that KBS in practice will be a potentially hazardous area.

The need for Decision Support remains urgent, and the potential savings both in health terms and in finance, promise to be substantial.

International Primary Care Computing
G.M. Hayes and N. Robinson (Editors)
Elsevier Science Publishers B.V. (North-Holland)
© IMIA, 1991

2.1   DECISION SUPPORT SYSTEMS IN PRIMARY CARE

R. Engelbrecht

Gesellschaft für Strahlen- und Umweltforschung mbH München Institut für
Medizinische Informatik und Systemforschung Ingolstädter Landstr. 1 8042 Neuherberg

Introduction

The goal of medical informatics is to enhance the quality of care with techniques of systems analysis, systems design and information processing. For the different areas of health care the International Medical Informatics Association (IMIA) has established working groups, e.g. WG5 for primary/ambulatory care. During the last working conference of WG5 in 1985 some topics were discussed in the fields of new technologies, networking, standardization in communication, medical records and expert systems in medicine (XPSM). During the past five years the computer technology has developed tremendously and influenced some areas of health care delivery. So it seems to be necessary to look at the expectations, recommendations and hopes of this workshop and to revise them for the field of decision support and knowledge based systems.

Statements from the Working Conference 1985

The presentations and results of the IMIA working conference 1985 are available in 2 volumes [9,10] and should be summarized briefly. The concluding remarks given by Peter L. Reichertz [11] are valid up till today:
"New technologies penetrate into the various sectors of ambulatory care. It is no question that the computer already plays an important role, though its influence is not yet ubiquitous. It is evident that this practice of general and ambulatory medicine needs further analysis in order to comprehend its decision making process and complexity. Before this is not done in a sufficient way, expert systems remain a subject for research and will not become a product of practical value. However, possible future applications can easily be imagined."

The workshop on expert systems XPSM [12] and some of the actual work presented may be followed up in a few paragraphs. The questions discussed in 1985 are shown in quotation marks:

"Why do we need research in KBS in primary care?"
The reasons are still valid: quality assurance, better treatment and equity of treatment. The statement "Expert systems research represents one of the core areas of medical informatics and demands cooperation between physicians and informaticians" is the key to a new German federal research programme MEDWIS (MEDizinische WISsensbasen = medical knowledge bases) which has just been started.

"What type of XPSM do we need?"
Main emphasis was seen in distributing existing knowledge for diagnosis, therapy and triage and this could also be a task for international cooperation today and in the future.
"In what area should we have XPSM?"
There was no area of primary care excluded, but integration into existing systems and the communication between systems were indicated as problem areas. This leads to ideas about cooperative KBS in the future which is a research task especially in an application like general medicine covering several medical disciplines.

"Evaluation and requirements for certification"
Evaluation of XPSM was seen as verification and assessment like conventional information systems. The validation of the knowledge base is quite a different new task and there are no standards available yet.

There were some systems for decision support in primary care presented and discussed at the working conference [4, 13, 14]. A follow up and new status report takes some effort and should be done separately. In this context only typical developments should be discussed briefly.

The XPSM SPHINX [4] was tested during an evaluation study by 40 GPs using Minitel [1], the French videotex system. It has shown its usefulness but also its limitation resulting from the knowledge base and technical environment.

The drug information system SMA [13] has by now entered the commercial market and is used as a supplement for pharmacy and doctors' office systems, a dedicated system for drug monitoring with its own patient data base [5] and as a tool for epidemiological studies [6].

The system ELIAS [14] has chosen the other way. Presented in 1985 as a system for primary care physicians and by now in commercial use it has been completed by a knowledge based module for quality assurance using the critiquing paradigm [7].

General Trends - results from technology assessment

There were 2 studies in 1986/87 TAES 86 [8, 3] and 1988/89 TAES 88 to assess the potential benefits as well as risks of expert systems in medicine (XPSM) in the temporal framework of the next ten to fifteen years, which was done for the German parliament. People working in the field were asked in questionnaires and in personal interviews to give their opinion about "chances and risks" of XPSM. The results of the assessment should help to identify lines of action that could promote the chances and prevent the disadvantages of medical XPSM.
The study brought results concerning the influence of expert systems on

- quality of care

- costs of care

- working structure and environment

- relationship physician/patient

- juridical and ethical implications.

There are some information retrieval systems, e.g. MEDIS [2], but few ESM which run through all stages of development and are in a practical application. But there is a growing tendency compared to a study done by Kulikowski and TAES 86 in 1983 and between both studies: TAES 86 and TAES 88. More than half the systems are in an experimental or design stage.

Legend:

MRU	**Medical research unit**
WUH	**Medical ward of a university hospital**
FUH	**Functional unit of a university hospital**
WGH	**Medical ward of a general hospital**
FGH	**Functional unit of a general hospital**
PC	**Ambulatory/primary care**
PH	**Public Health Service**
OTH	**Other institutions**

Fig. 1: Settings in which Expert Systems are applied Source: TAES88 (number of systems = 58. [2] multiple checks possible).

A consequence of this development status is the distribution of settings where ESM are applied or tested (Fig. 1). The systems are mostly implemented in the neighbourhood of the developers which is usually for systems under development. Different from this result are the expectations of the usage of ESM in the year 2000. Nearly the same number of systems is expected in the wards of a general hospital as in a doctor's office. Compared to the increased usage of EDP systems in general in both settings during the last 15 years this might be realistic and should have a deep effect in the future.

The final part of the questionnaire dealt with a set of theses on which the interviewed persons could agree or reject the statement. Again it should be mentioned that most of the 67 participants in this mailing survey were developers or 'experts' in the field. 98% of all 43 participants who answered agreed to the statement "xps will enhance the quality of care". The enhancement of quality of care by "more precise drug information to avoid side effects and interactions" was agreed by 97%. On the next rank there were ease of quality assurance and improvement of medical services by more standardization with 83% agreement. More sceptical ratings were given with about 50% for "communication enhancement" and "better coordination in the treatment process".

XPSM should be able to increase the transparency and give assistance to the different processes in the health care system. This quality enhancement is the reason for money saving in some cases but not in all. Thus the answers to the costs of care seem to be realistic. Nearly three quarters of all participants agreed that XPSM will enable a more specific, faster, and better diagnostic and therapeutical process. The drug prescriptions were mentioned with 90%.

The general conclusion could be drawn that the increasing of quality of care decreases the costs. But this is too simple. The most remarkable statement given may be seen in the substitution of clinical care by outpatient care. This may influence the costs, but it influences more the structure of the health care system. Clinical knowledge applied in primary care could be able to give the general practitioners a greater competence and in that way a greater effectiveness. But this is depending on the type of health care system. There might be differences in systems with strict separation of primary and secondary care as in Germany or systems like the US one, where physicians have beds in hospitals and in this way are getting clinical experience.

Influence of Medical Expert Systems on Treatment

The 1988 technology assessment study was completed by two case studies. Firstly there was the application of the interaction component of the drug information system SMA on representative medication data. This data were provided by the MI (myocardial infarction) registry and a cross sectional study of the MONICA project Augsburg. One result was that about 25% of the MI-patients had the risk of a drug interaction in their medication before the MI and 53% after the MI. A detailed analysis may give some hints for the use of this type of monitoring system in daily practice.

The second study was dedicated to the problem of patient/ physician interaction. The test field was provided by the hospital Munich Bogenhausenwhere. The personal computer assisted consultation system CAMIT was used for diabetic patients. Forty patients from the diabetes center Bogenhausen were asked about their relationship to the role of a computer during the treatment. The results are encouraging. None of the patients was disturbed by use of a computer at the physician's. 92% agreed with the statement "If computers are useful for physicians then my family physician should also have one." This gives a clear mandate to medical informatics.

Summary

Some of the above mentioned research tasks are described too briefly and need a discussion. This is done mainly in the different countries where working or socialist groups on XPSM or artificial intelligence exist. Another place is the international meetings like MEDINFO, MIE and AIME. But also the European community has developed a program called AIM (Advanced Informatics in Medicine) with many relationships to XPSM and some to primary care, e.g. the projects EURODIABETA, GAMES, KAVAS and PRECISE. Especially, PRECISE is dealing with the consulting situation of physicians. There is no question that new techniques have their impact on the situation at the work place. In general the chances are seen in higher qualified workload and more time for the patient. But this section is very speculative and there are a lot of consequences drawn from the experience during the ongoing process of automatization in the industry and administration. Results could be gained from the user centered analysis within PRECISE.

In any case the tendency to assist in routine situations like creating a diagnostic plan is to be seen and the effect might be that XPS will take over a portion of relatively simple tasks and give time for creative and high quality tasks or more time for the patients. There is no doubt amongst most interviewees that a loss of jobs is not to be expected.

During the interviews most of the experts associated positive expectations with an introduction of XPSM in the near future. But they did not neglect the risks which may occur. A discussion concerning the introduction of a new technology was never so engaged in that early stage of development as it was in the field of expert systems in medicine. From the standpoint of the developer this is fruitful and enables the physician to discuss his problems in other structures and context. The reflection of an interdisciplinary discussion between physicians and informaticians are the main benefits of XPSM from a scientific standpoint of view and will have influence on medicine and informatics.

References

[1]   Botti, G., Joubert, M., Fieschi, DF, Proudhon, H., Fieschi, M., 1989, Experimental Use of the Medical Expert System SPHINX by General Practitioners: Results and Analysis In: MEDINFO '89 Proceedings, B. Barber, C. Cao, D. Quin, G. Wagner (Eds.), North Holland, 1989, p.67-71

[2]   Collen, M.F., Flagle, Ch.D., 1985, Full-Text Medical Literature Retrieval by Computer - A Pilot Test, JAMA, 254, 19, 1985, p. 2768 - 2774

[3]   Engelbrecht, R.Potthoff, P., Schwefel, D., 1987, Expert Systems in Medicine - Results from a Technology Assessment Study, In: DIAC 87, CPSR, Seattle/USA, 1987, p. 125 - 134

[4]   Engelbrecht, R., Rothemund, M., 1987, Workshop on Expert Systems and User Needs resp. Patient Records, in 10, p.196-198

[5]   Engelbrecht, R., Schaaf, R.,Scholz, W., 1987, Pharmaceutical Consultation System for Physicians and Pharmacists - Basis for an Expert System, Proceedings MIE '87, A. Serio, R. O'Moore, A. Tardini, F.H. Roger, 1987, p.1106-1115

[6]   Engelbrecht, R., Schaaf, R., Lewis, M., 1989, Assistance in Medical Treatment and Treatment Analysis with an Interactive Drug Consultation System In: MEDINFO '89 Proceedings, B. Barber, C. Cao, D. Quin, G. Wagner (Eds.), North Holland, 1989, p.

[7]   van der Lei, J., van der Heijden, p., Boon, W.M., 1989, Critiquing Expert Critiques: Issues for the Development of computer-based Monitoring in Primary Care In: MEDINFO '89 Proceedings, B. Barber, C. Cao, D. Quin, G. Wagner (Eds.), North Holland, 1989, p.106-110

[8]   Potthoff, P., Schwefel, D. Rothemund, M. Engelbrecht, R., van Eimeren, W., 1988,Expert Systems in Medicine, Int. J. of Technology Assessment in Health Care 4, 1988, p. 121-133

[9]   Reichertz, P.L., Engelbrecht, R., Piccolo, U, 1987, System Analysis of Ambulatory Care in Selected Countries, Lecture Notes in Medical Informatics, P.L. Reichertz, D.A.B. Lindberg (Eds.), Springer, 29, 1987,

[10]   Reichertz, P.L., Engelbrecht, R., Piccolo, U, 1987, Present Status of Computer Support in Ambulatory Care, Lecture Notes in Medical Informatics, P.L. Reichertz, D.A.B. Lindberg (Eds.), Springer, 30, 1987,

[11]   Reichertz, P.L., Concluding Considerations, in [10], p. 199-209

[12]   Rothemund, M., Engelbrecht, R.:, 1987, Expert Systems in Primary Care. in [10], p. 75-85

[13]   Schaaf, R., Wassermann, G., Engelbrecht, R., Scholz, W. , 1987 Medical Treatment Assistance with an Interactive Drug Information System, p. 159 - 164

[14]   Westerhof, H.P., Boon, W.M., Cromme, P.V.M., van Bemmel, J.H., 1987, in [10], p.1-10

International Primary Care Computing
G.M. Hayes and N. Robinson (Editors)
Elsevier Science Publishers B.V. (North-Holland)
© IMIA, 1991

2.2 MEDICAL DECISION SUPPORT

Andrzej Glowinski

Clinical Research Fellow, Imperial Cancer Research Fund Laboratories, P.O. BOX NO. 123, Lincolns Inn Fields, London

Introduction

Medical decision support can, for our purposes, be divided into two types. The first is concerned with supporting the formulation of medical policies, largely by gathering and analysing population-based data; the second deals with clinical decisions, helping the physician to apply medical knowledge, including these policies, to the care of the individual patient. This discussion concentrates on the second of these.

Clinical decision support systems have evolved considerably since they were first proposed over two decades ago. Recent designs have matured significantly, and the view of workers in the area is that systems will move from the laboratory to the clinical work place in increasing numbers in the next decade (for example the TAES86 and TAES88 studies) (Engelbrecht et al, 1987). However, despite the potential for improving the quality of care, a number of factors will greatly affect the acceptance of clinical decision support by individual physicians and the medical community as a whole.

Here, five topics that may be important in the introduction of clinical decision support systems for use by physicians are considered: the role of the decision support system; the style of support; the choice of decision support techniques, and how they are applied; various aspects of integration of the system; and how the system may be appropriately evaluated. No attempt has been made to be exhaustive; this discussion is intended to be a starting point for the workshop.

The Role of the Decision Support System

Specifying what is required of software presumes that its role is well defined. During development of decision support systems, their role often seems to be relegated to the background, only to appear glaringly neglected as the system migrates from computer laboratory through field tests to the clinic. Most medical decision support systems have been developed within hospital or specialist environments, which differ considerably from primary care. Questions such as "Which decisions do physicians require help with?" and "Where does uncertainty arise?" are of prime importance, but too frequently ignored. Alan Rector (Rector et al, 1989) provides evidence that primary care physicians experience uncertainty very frequently, even with commonplace problems, and Toomas Timpka (Timpka and Arborelius, 1990) has illustrated the variety of dilemmas that GPs encounter.

Further questions must be answered before appropriate decision support can be devised: does the uncertainty experienced lead to suboptimal choices? (the doctor adopting, for instance, "wait and see" strategies which can lead to unnecessary delays. There is considerable evidence that this is the case, particularly in the management of malignant disease). On the other hand, many decisions pose no difficulties,and hence require no assistance. What do physicians do well, and when are mistakes made? Unless the answers to these questions are known, the design is likely to be inappropriate.

The role of the system vis a vis the individual physician forms only a part of the picture. The organisation of health care and its delivery will fundamentally affect this role, irrespective of the technical performance of the system. Whatever positive attributes the system possesses it must fit in with the way health care is delivered. Frequently, computer systems are only occasionally accessed by the intended group of users, and other members of the health care team do most of the work - this is certainly the case for many computerised record systems. Is decision support likely to be any different?

The potential consequences the introduction of decision support could have, both on the organisation and delivery of services and on the care of individuals, should not be underestimated, and require careful monitoring.

The potential consequences of introducing decision support are great, both on the care of individuals and on the organisation and delivery of services. The hope is that care may be improved, for instance with fewer unnecessary operations and a lower incidence of drug side effects, and that costs may be reduced. However, these effects are not guaranteed: careful monitoring of changes in the outcome of treatment and costs are vital.

The Style of Support

The way in which help in making decisions is provided governs how useful and acceptable the system is, irrespective of the content of the help provided. What sort of help would be most acceptable? Helping the physician to "repair" a decision that appears to have gone wrong, or recover from a "breakdown" of the decision making process (e.g. because of a lack of knowledge or an impasse being reached), may be far more useful than making a complete decision de novo. To do this effectively, a range of support facilities is needed, allowing the user to determine the starting and end points and the nature of the information provided (Glowinski et al, 1989).

But how can such support be delivered in practice? The balance of control between user and machine has perceptibly swung away from the early computer-dominated, prescriptive style towards more user-centred and passive systems. To an extent this change results from some of the discomforting effects that machine controlled interaction can have. Universally adopting the user-centred style would, however, fail to acknowledge that doctors make a wide range of decisions: it is unlikely that all of these demand the same balance of control between physician and machine. Some tasks may be best served by a background

"watchdog", others by providing information at the request of the user, or guiding the physician, whilst at times the system may appropriately prompt without being asked.
More studies are needed to determine the most effective style of information provision. Undoubtedly, a complex combination of factors is at work: amongst others, the nature of the decision, the environment the decision is made in, and the individual doctor's preferences will all turn out to be important.

Decision Support Techniques: Choice and Application

Much has been written about the various techniques that are used in decision support systems. These range over the use of databases (eg relational algebra), quantitative handling of uncertainty (eg Bayes theorem, certainty factors), and symbolic inference techniques (eg those derived from artificial intelligence). However, relatively little attention has been paid to how these techniques are chosen and used in a particular application.

Although many of the techniques are formalised and their use fully specified, some are only gradually being characterised and formalised. There is a tendency, particularly in the realm of expert systems, to use even well understood techniques in rather ad hoc ways, often without detailed descriptions of how they behave or perform in that application (Fox et al, 1990). As a result, it may be difficult to understand or predict how a system will function, a factor that inevitably leads to a loss of confidence.

Many of the techniques employed are quite general in nature, but are often inextricably mixed with domain specific information within the application. This severely limits the scope for an extension of functionality or expansion of the medical content, integration with other systems (see below) or - perhaps most important - updating the medical information, without rewriting the whole system. This is impractical; the way in which techniques are used can have significant implications for the demand on time and resources.

We can ask several questions about the techniques themselves and how they are used in the particular application:-

Are the techniques used general, or are they specific to the application?

Have the techniques used been formalised?

Are they used in a standard manner in the application?

Is their use in the software formally specified?

How have they been evaluated?

Is the choice appropriate to the problem being tackled?

Too often systems are devised where the technique is chosen before the goals of the system are fully defined.

Integration of the system

A decision support system has to be well integrated to function smoothly. Integration can occur along three axes: across the domain, across different types of support, and with other systems.

Primary care is not easily separable into medical specialties. Problems often transcend specialties, so the information provided must not be constrained by these boundaries. Integration across the medical domain is vital for the system to fit into the everyday practice of the general practitioner. Decisions are seldom taken in any strictly predetermined order, as might be suggested by the various descriptions of the consultation, such as the medical model: history, investigation, diagnosis, treatment, follow-up (Fox and Rector, 1982).

As a complement to integration across the domain is the need to integrate the different types and levels of support, so that the system can immediately respond to the user's information requirements as they change during the evolution of a decision. Requests for more detail, checklists, opinions and so on should not each require a fresh start, nor should there be a limitation on the order in which the requests can be made.

Information technology is having an increasing impact in the medical workplace, decision support systems being perhaps the most recent addition. Integration of "office systems" is a major activity, and it is natural that decision support systems should be part of this. Developers often build their prototypes in isolation, but transfer to the consultation room without bearing in mind that other computerised systems will be present reduces the usability of the finished product. In particular, computerised patient records, laboratory data services, and other decision support information sources (such as those supporting the formulation of medical policies) must be fully accessible.

Evaluation

Evaluation of decision support systems is complex. Planning the evaluation may be simplified, however, if appropriate tests are chosen for the various components of the system. Both the design and implementation can be subdivided into parts that can be individually examined: overall goals, roles, compatibility with existing health care organisation; the interface, inference mechanism, etc.

"Performance" cannot be characterised by a single parameter, so an appropriate range of measures has to be identified. Too frequently, the single attribute of "accuracy" has been used, especially in the case of first generation diagnostic expert systems. For general practice measures of how complete and relevant the information is, and how accessible and robust the operation of the system, are just as important.

Testing may be broadly divided into laboratory evaluations (during system development) and field tests. The process may be compared with that of testing a new drug (Wyatt, 1987). Laboratory evaluations of the components of the system allow comparisons and choices to be made at an early stage, for instance of the techniques to be employed (eg O'Neil et al,

1990). Once confident that the system works in the laboratory, field tests can be undertaken. These may result in modifications to the system, but these should not be drastic. However, there are too many stories of high performance systems remaining unused because they do not do what the doctor wants in an acceptable way, to allow us to be complacent about the quality of current evaluations.

Evaluation cannot be confined to the performance of the system in isolation. It will be part of a clinical environment, and have effects on and be affected by the organisation of health care delivery. These effects may have implications for the quality of care provided and the demand on resources, so must be examined in addition to function of the system in its own right.

Conclusions

Before medical decision support systems can successfully make the transition from a research environment to everyday clinical use it must be recognised that this is not simply a process of becoming technically more mature. The primary care environment in particular differs substantially from the hospital specialties, with its own requirements and constraints, and attention must be directed towards coping with these before decision support can become acceptable to the physician working as part of a complex health care system.

References

Engelbrecht R, Potthoff P, Schwefel D (1987) "Expert systems in medicine - results from a technology assessment study. In: DIAC87, CPSR, Seattle, USA, 1987, pp 125-134

Fox J, Glowinski A J, O'Neil M J (1990) "Reliable and reusable tools for medical knowledge based systems". To appear in J Talmon and J Fox (eds) Proceedings of the Conference on AI in Medicine, COMAC-BME, Maastricht, 1989. Springer-Verlag

Fox J, Rector A L (1982) "Expert Systems for Primary Medical Care?". Automedica, 4, pp 123-130

Glowinski A J, O'Neil M J, Fox J (1989) "Design of a generic information system and it application to primary care". In: Hunter J, Cookson J, Wyatt J (eds.): Proceedings of the Second European Conference on Artificial Intelligence in Medicine. Lecture Notes in Medical Informatics 38, pp 221-233, Springer-Verlag

O'Neil M, Glowinski A J, Fox J (1990) "Evaluating and validating very large knowledge based systems" Medical Informatics (in press).

Rector A L, Brooke J B, Sheldon M G, Newton P D (1989) "An analysis of uncertainty in British general practice: implications of a preliminary survey". In: Hunter J, Cookson J, Wyatt J (eds.): Proceedings of the

32

Second European Conference on Artificial Intelligence in Medicine.
Lecture Notes in Medical Informatics 38, pp 259-268, Springer-Verlag

Timpka T, Arborelius E (1990) "The GP's dilemmas: a study of   knowledge
need and use during health care consultations". Methods of
Information in Medicine 29, pp 23-29

Wyatt J (1987) "The evaluation of clinical decision support   systems: a
discussion of the methodology used in the ACORN project".   In: Fox J,
Fieschi M, Engelbrecht R (eds.): Proceedings of the First European
Conference on Artificial Intelligence in Medicine. Lecture Notes in
Medical Informatics 33, pp 15-24, Springer-Verlag

International Primary Care Computing
G.M. Hayes and N. Robinson (Editors)
Elsevier Science Publishers B.V. (North-Holland)
© IMIA, 1991

3 CODING

Chairman, W A Nowlan

Medical Informatics Group Dept. of Computer Science Manchester University Oxford Road Manchester M19 9PL

Presenter, R Weeks

9 Upper Brighton Road Surbiton Surrey KT6 6LQ

Discussant, S Shepherd

Lawrence Hill Health Centre, Hassell Drive, Lawrence Hill, Bristol BS2 0AN UK

Rapporteur, M Bainbridge

The Surgery Hexton Road Barton Beds.

Introduction

The workshop discussion focused primarily on the current state of coding within health-care systems. The participants presented many perspectives on the problem, derived for example from primary and secondary care, or a clinical versus a resource managerial orientation. This great diversity of opinions and specific needs was a manifestation of two important principles -

> all the components of a health service need to interact with information systems and the techniques used to represent information within such a system are of central importance

> there is potentially a large range of uses and purposes for such information, but those uses may be heavily influenced by the choice of representation

An analysis of the sources of this variation is essential if we are to understand those needs and identify workable solutions to a set of fundamental informatics problems. I shall attempt to outline briefly several general themes which I feel emerged during the discussion, and thereby help in disentangling some of the many compounded ideas.

Language

The term representation has been used in preference to "coding". Some of the difficulties that arise during debates on "coding" are undoubtedly due to a confusion over terminology. In general "coding" compounds the idea of coding systems with their uses. This is a mistake.

At least three different interpretations can be identified:

- the act of creating a coding system such as ICD-9, or the system itself;
- the act of turning a medical statement into a code;
- the act of generating an electronic medical record.

An adequate coding system is necessary if medical statements are to be coded and included within an electronic medical record. But a medical record is a complex document and much more than the sum of its parts, or a simple collection of "codes". Thus an adequate coding system, judged by criteria such as completeness, does not in itself guarantee its usability and ensure its correct use. Furthermore the correct use of the system is a necessary but not sufficient prerequisite to a complete medical record. It is essential to identify not only what a coding system can achieve but also what it cannot. Additional mechanisms or structures will be required to specify the complete record and ensure the correct use of the coding system. The term coding also implies a strong reference to the code numbers themselves, which are really of secondary importance to the underlying conceptual structure. In order to avoid such confusions it may be preferable to use the term representation to refer to the abstract structure.

Purpose

Probably the most serious source of divergent opinions is derived from the multiplicity of purposes for which a coding system is to be used. In particular there appears to be a central tension between the use of a coding system:

- to keep patient records for the clinical management of the individual
- for collecting, analysing and interpreting aggregated data

Different groups place unequal emphasis on these views and it would be easy to adopt stereotypes. It is also common however for a single group to wish for both views. The clinician will use information to care for the individual patient, but at another time will want to audit his or her activity and performance for a larger group of patients.

A complete electronic medical record requires a comprehensive, highly expressive system, and it was suggested during the discussion that a nomenclature rather than a classification was more appropriate. It may also be necessary however to accommodate expressions of uncertainty, and provisional diagnoses, as well as concepts such as "patient's reason for encounter". The clinicians were particularly concerned with the need to record diagnoses as a synthesis of their ideas and the basis for planning management. They were quite willing to accept that the diagnosis may later change as the management evolved, but that it is unacceptable to restrict coding to "absolute truth" or only signs and symptoms as representing the raw material of the true diagnosis. It was correctly pointed out during the discussion that medical records are full of diagnoses and opinions that subsequently are proved to be mistaken, but that does not imply it was incorrect to record them at the time.

The aggregation of data requires some form of classified or organized structure. As has already been argued by Dr Shepherd, it is vital to exercise caution in the collection and analysis of aggregated data, particularly across organizational boundaries. When aggregating data a highly expressive and detailed system may lead to the inconsistent recording of data, and incorrect deductions. A coding system by itself cannot prevent such errors. This requires the evaluation and verification of both the system and its use, within the appropriate setting.

When data is aggregated there is always a purpose in mind, and this gives rise to yet further conflicts. The needs of a manager may be quite different from those of the public health expert, and they may wish to aggregate the data in quite different ways. Information systems will need to support this diversity of uses, and if they are not to fragment, they will require a core representation. These sorts of differing requirements are the basis of many arguments over coding. They are really arguments over classification, but reaffirm that there is no single purpose for a coding system. In this respect a discussion took place over the current use of the Read Clinical Classification within the UK, and it was suggested that many debates could be resolved if it was renamed the Read Clinical Nomenclature.

Conclusions

This workshop tackled a difficult and complex topic. The expression of so many opinions and needs in itself serves to highlight the existence of several central problems. Probably the main challenge facing workers in this field is to identify those very issues and mark the boundaries of competence of the current methodologies. We must be critical in our use of coding systems, have a clarity of purpose when using them, and understand the limitations of any system in order to avoid abuse and erroneous conclusions.

In looking to the future it is essential to establish the basis for the extension and refinement of current methodologies. This requires three areas of work:

- theoretical research and development of representation systems
- their implementation and evaluation in practical systems
- education of both medical and computer professionals

"Coding" can only be sensibly addressed within the broader task of representing medical information within computer systems. This is an absolute prerequisite to the development of systems capable of meeting the growing expectations and needs of clinicians and managers.

International Primary Care Computing
G.M. Hayes and N. Robinson (Editors)
Elsevier Science Publishers B.V. (North-Holland)
© IMIA, 1991

3.1 PAN EUROPEAN CLINICAL CLASSIFICATION

Dr S G Shepherd

Lawrence Hill Health Centre, Hassell Drive, Lawrence Hill, Bristol BS2 0AN

Introduction

There is no need, in this setting, to set out the arguments in favour of a Pan European Clinical Classification. Information Technology has given us the means to acquire unprecedented insight into clinical data on a grand scale. However like any powerful tool Information Technology also gives us the opportunity to increase on an equally grand scale the size and scope of the mistakes we can make.

We are on the threshold of a computerised network of primary care physicians across Europe. To maximise this opportunity we must have a clinical classification that is capable of exploiting the opportunity to the full.

There is a real danger that we may, especially in the UK in a rush to create a Pan European Clinical Classification, adopt the quickest solution and not necessarily the most appropriate.

How Much Data is Needed?

One of the principal aims in gathering health care data is the evaluation of the benefits and costs of health care. Information Technology allows us to aggregate a vast quantity of data to this end. However we may aggregate nonsense as effortlessly as we aggregate fact.

We need to understand the data we collect. One of the meanings of "understand" in the Oxford English Dictionary is to "take for granted". When we "understand" the term another doctor has recorded we may be simply taking for granted that he and we mean the same thing. There is evidence to the contrary.

Consider gastritis, dyspepsia and indigestion. These are not synonyms. Can we be sure that even all the doctors in this room use these terms invariably consistently? If they do not what are we adding up when we aggregate their computerised practice returns?

If doctors were only allowed to code that the patient did or did not have cancer we might reasonably expect that the codes would be used consistently even across Europe. However as the number of codes rises so the opportunity for inconsistent use rises exponentially.

There is a need for an agreed body of medical concepts and terms for these are the building blocks of a classification. If we do not agree on what these terms mean then any structure we build will be inherently flawed. Having agreed them we must then also ensure that the relevant health care providers know the agreed meaning.

It is a monumental folly to aggregate data collected at a level of detail beyond the level which we have defined and agreed.

False aggregated information is much worse than no aggregated information.

We must not fall into the familiar medical trap where having found we can measure something we do measure it, and then because we have measured it we attribute significance to it.

So it is with Blood Pressure. If the Medical Research Council is right and that we need to control the blood pressure in 850 patients to prevent one of them having a stroke, it is clear that, as far as the prevention of strokes is concerned, we are measuring the wrong thing. It may be easy to measure blood pressure but it may be a waste of time.

So it may be with codes. It may be possible to allocate 250,000 codes to codify the whole of medicine. Having allocated the codes, we use them and we count them and because we have counted them we attribute significance to them. But what have we actually achieved? Like blood pressure it is easy to measure but is it worthwhile?

How Many Codes are Needed?

Clearly a mere handful of codes would be too crude. But for how many can we have an agreed meaning and, in addition, be sure that all health care providers observe the meaning consistently?

We can look at the prevalence of diseases seen by European family doctors. There are some 250 diseases with a prevalence of over 5 per 1000 persons per annum. There are about 500 between 1 and 5 per 1000 persons per annum.

Even at a frequency as rare as less than 1 per 100,000 persons per annum there are only a modest 4,000 diseases to be seen in Primary Care. What is the value of coding, in Primary Care, these rarities unless we can be certain that we are using even the first 250 terms consistently?

It is inescapable that the greater the number of codes the more closely packed they become and the subtler are the differences between them and the opportunities for inconsistent use rise.

Some will argue that too few codes force the doctor to use inappropriate codes. This problem is not a function of the number of codes but of their precision. Forcing occurs when the doctor is faced with too precise codes rather than too few codes.

It is not the number of codes that matters at all. It is what they mean to each health care provider that determines their usefulness and if they mean different things then their usefulness is substantially limited.

We should only count what is meaningful. It is a fallacy that the more specific the code, the more reliable it becomes. The opposite is true.

Fine Detail

If we have fewer codes how are we to record fine detail? The precision of codes must match the purpose for which the code is required and no more. That principle will determine the number any health care provider needs.

Provided renal physicians agree on the meanings of codes they may use them and aggregate them. But it would be foolish to permit GPs or gynaecologists to use those codes unless they too understood fully the agreed meaning of the code.

If a GP wishes to record finer detail free text comment will suffice. The free text will not be aggregated by computer and will protect against inconsistent codes rendering the aggregation meaningless.

Coders may deride free text. We are all aware of its limits. But to seek to code every variation and every nuance of clinical care offers unlimited scope for inconsistent coding and meaningless aggregation.

What Data Should be Coded?

One of the principal aims of gathering health care data is the evaluation of the benefits and costs of health care and medical interventions in particular.

Analysis of diagnoses and symptoms alone simply does not explain the variations in health needs, provisions, interventions and outcomes. To understand health care we must capture all aspects of the patients' transactions with health services including patients' motivations and expectations, their functional status and how these are changed by the medical interventions.

The classification needs to encompass the reason for encounter, severity of symptoms, objective findings, diagnosis, functional status, intervention, and outcome.

Functional status indicators measure change in function of patients over time judged by both the patient and the doctor. The number of hip operations done in the NHS last year tells us something. The numbers of people who returned to work, who regained mobility, who returned to independent living, or who did not and became dependent on others after a hip operation tells us dramatically more.

What we record is much more important than how much we record.

Compatibility

For the future in Europe compatibility with ICD.10 is an essential prerequisite and has been explicitly stated as such by AIM.

However conversion from one classification to another is rarely straightforward. There may be an exact correlation in both directions for some codes. However the code in one classification may be more specific or less specific than the nearest code in the other classification. Or the two codes may be incompatible, one not being found in the other classification at all.

If a classification claims to be compatible with another there should be published evidence to verify the claim.

The importance of a detailed rigorous approach with open publication of the results cannot be over emphasised. For once a choice is made in favour of a particular classification the possibility to compare results with another is limited.

The European Dimension

What has been stated above applies within one country. Expanding across Europe adds a vast new dimension.

Cultural differences within the same country are considerable. Medical terms and concepts are intimate and personal and as a result these concepts vary over even short distances.

The aim of translation is not semantic but conceptual and cultural to capture the clinically relevant translation of the clinical entity. It is not the words but the meaning that matters. We must be extraordinarily careful not to oversimplify.

A symptom group in the UK might be labelled Gastritis. We do not really know that there is inflammation of the stomach lining but we have grown accustomed to this concept. In, perhaps, Italy the same symptom group might be labelled Choledyskinesia - impaired motility of the gall bladder. Do we know with certainty which is the more accurate pathological description?

If we translate these two terms into each other's language they will not be perceived as the same though the patient's story was identical.

What does Coronary insufficiency mean in different parts of Europe?

In West Germany hypotension is a disease. Many Germans are treated for this disease of low blood pressure. How are we to translate that conceptually and culturally into English medicine?

Are we any wiser to be "treating" glue ear with oral decongestants? What would a Portuguese doctor make of glue ear?

It is naive to think that by translating language we are also translating clinical entities.

What is the Starting Point?

It is essential that the evolution of any classification is based on evaluation and published data. It is impossible to overstate this point. If we do not we will simply create the Pan European Clinical Illusion.

That a classification is in use by a large number of doctors is no guarantee of its effectiveness and is certainly no substitute for scientific evaluation.

There is only one Primary Care classification that has published organisational principles, that has evolved through consistent academic research with published data, that has evaluated the usefulness of the codes, that has published compatibility with ICD.10 and that is designed to capture the whole of the Primary Care transaction. That is the International Classification for Primary Care (ICPC). ICPC is at least a candidate for Europe.

ICPC has a limited number of codes but they produce an almost overwhelming wealth of data. Because the classification has been thoroughly evaluated that wealth of data may be aggregated and analysed in confidence rather than in hope.

In the ICPC Transition project, for instance, 100,000 reasons for encounter were evaluated by 100 providers in 12 countries.

A current ICPC project is to video consultations, interview patients after the consultation and compare the video and the patient's perceptions with the doctor's coded reason for encounter to evaluate over or under interpretation. This is the right way to move forward, in certainty.

In September 1989 an ICPC European Community Workshop met at Padua with representatives of 12 European Counties. The overwhelmingly agreed need was for a joint meeting of all the translators to allow a code by code discussion and translation to establish the clinically relevant translation rather than merely the semantic translation. Such a meeting is to take place in London in September 1990 organised by Update Computers.

This will provide the first European clinical, rather than merely semantic, translation of a primary care classification.

Summary

Europe needs to develop a Clinical Classification to exploit to the full the opportunities offered by Information Technology.

The need is for a classification that is:

- powerful enough for the opportunity before us

- subject to a continuing rigorous published evaluation of the codes and their usefulness

- capable of capturing the whole health care transaction

- compatible with ICD.10 on the basis of published evidence

- available in a Europe wide clinical translation

Europe should not adopt a classification that does not fulfil these criteria. However pressing the need, however much we want a European classification, the wrong classification, once adopted will be difficult and expensive to replace.

International Primary Care Computing
G.M. Hayes and N. Robinson (Editors)
Elsevier Science Publishers B.V. (North-Holland)
© IMIA, 1991

4 SCREENING

4.1 Improving the Effectiveness of Screening in General Practice

Mike Fitter and Paul Norman

MRC/ESRC Social & Applied Psychology Unit, University of Sheffield, Sheffield S10 2TN UK

Abstract

This paper examines different computer-based methods of inviting patients for screening in General Practice. Its aim is to identify the pros and cons of various methods from the perspective of the practice (comprehensive, cost-effective screening), and from the perspective of the patient (acceptable and reassuring without undue interference).

A comparison of the CALL method (a letter sent to all patients in the target groups) and the OPPORTUNISTIC method (a personal invitation made when the patient attends at the surgery) is reported. Preliminary results indicate that opportunistic screening is more efficient for the practice and more convenient for patients. The call method can be superior for sustaining a high level of invitations. However, the effectiveness of Call depends crucially on the contents and style of the invitation letter.

To achieve comprehensive and cost effective screening within an appropriate timescale requires a combination of both methods, designed to meet the specific needs of the practice and its population.

Introduction

Preventive screening in General Practice in the UK is on the increase. Following the Government's White Paper 'Promoting Better Health' [1], the new contract for GPs states that GPs will be paid by how effectively they screen and provide preventive services to their registered patients.

It is generally recognised that the computer will be a necessary tool of General Practice, to administer the service efficiently, and to monitor and audit performance [2].

One aim of the research is to investigate and promote realistic ways of using a computer to provide a preventive service. Another aim is to examine the quality and impact of the service from the clients' (patients') perspective.

In this paper we examine the first step in this process, the initial screening of patients, and evaluate two commonly used methods of inviting patients to attend for a health check. These methods are 'Call' and 'Opportunistic' invitation.

By Call invitation we mean that the practice uses a patient register to identify and Call patients in the target group (for example, by sending a letter). By Opportunistic invitation we mean waiting until the patient visits the practice for whatever reason and then, if they are in the target group, taking the opportunity to invite them to be screened. Thus the essential difference between the two methods is who initiates the original contact from which the invitation arises (practice or patient). Of course there are many variations on the way each method can be delivered (what the letter says, how many follow-ups are sent, who makes an Opportunistic invite etc.) and some of these are discussed in this paper.

There are many studies which report on either attendance rates for a particular method (eg [3]) or changes in the proportion of patients for whom health measures are recorded as a result of a screening programme (eg [4]). However, it is difficult to draw any firm conclusions on the relative effectiveness of different invitation methods from these studies. To make such a comparison requires matching of practice and patient population characteristics, and this is best done by making comparisons within a practice.

Evaluation Criteria

The aim of the study is to compare the effectiveness of Call and Opportunistic invitation to health screening. The criteria of effectiveness are:

1. The coverage of the target population achieved, broken down by population characteristics (age, sex, social status, health beliefs etc.). We are particularly interested in the 'barriers' to attendance as perceived by patients.

2. The administrative cost of achieving the coverage, including clinical and administrative staff time and resources used.

3. The acceptability of the method to the patients, assessed by questionnaire (and interview for a subsample) immediately after the screening session. Acceptability includes assessment of patients' perceptions of the value and convenience of screening.

4. The acceptability of the method to the practice. In particular, PHCT and administrative staffs' views on the ease of administration, the ability to maintain a steady flow of patients, the appropriateness of invitations etc.

An Evaluation in one General Practice

Currently we are carrying out our research in three practices. This paper reports on the study in one of the practices and provides data and preliminary conclusions following the first 6 months of operation of the screening programme.

The practice is providing a screening programme to all of one GP's patients aged between 30 and 50 years (565 patients), carried out by a practice nurse. They are given a general health check, their lipid levels are measured, they have an opportunity to discuss any general health matters, and they are offered a tetanus injection if appropriate. Based on a protocol, if lipid levels are raised the patient is invited to enter a diet education and improvement programme. There is a 'basic' and an 'intense' programme. This latter comparison is part of a separate study which will be reported subsequently.

Research Design and Method

The 565 patients in the target population were randomly assigned to one of 3 groups:

> 189 patients in the Call group
>
> 190 patients in the Opportunistic group
>
> 186 patients in a control group (who will be screened 12 months later as part of the diet programme study).

Patients were sent a Health Questionnaire by post prior to invitation to be screened. This was to obtain basic information on social characteristics (employment status, social support available etc) and on patients' health beliefs, behaviours (smoking etc) and attitudes to health screening and preventive care. This information is being used to assess whether these patient characteristics predict attendance at the screening session and subsequent changes in behaviour and attitude.

Patients who did not return the questionnaire were sent a further copy. A total of 243 completed questionnaires were returned and an additional 17 were returned because of incorrect addresses. Removing the incorrect addresses from the sample, the overall response rate was 68%.

At the end of the screening session the patients were asked to complete a further questionnaire and return it to the researchers by post. This was to obtain patients' views on the session and on the way in which they were invited to it. We could thus compare patients' views on the two methods of invitation. A smaller sample of 11 patients were also given a tape recorded interview at this point to obtain more detailed views.

Principal steps in the procedure
1. Allocation of patients to experimental groups.

2. Postal distribution of Health Questionnaires to patients, and follow up of non-responders.

3. Tagging of the notes of patients in the Opportunistic group so that they could be identified and invited when visiting the practice.

4. Establishment of an appointment book for the health check clinic.

5. Checking and distribution of first month's batch of 60 computer produced invitation letters to patients in the Call group.

6. GP begins inviting 'tagged' patients to make an appointment for the health check clinic. A few patients are invited by the practice nurse or reception staff. (A 'quota' of 15 opportunistic invites per week is set).

7. Reception staff change or cancel appointments when requests are received.

8. Patients are screened and afterwards complete an evaluation questionnaire.

9. Data is recorded on invitations, changed appointments, attenders and non-attenders, patients asking to be excluded, or excluded by the GP, temporarily or indefinitely.

10. This data is used to continue selecting patients for invitation and to assess the effectiveness of the invitation methods.

11. Patients who DNA are written to by the practice nurse. If they fail to respond again they are phoned.

12. At the end of the trial, Opportunistic group patients who have not been invited are written to as a final 'sweep-up'.

Results from the first Six Months of the Trial

During the initial period of operation a total of 217 patients have been invited to attend the health check clinic. The results below present a preliminary analysis of the data.

TABLE 1. Attendance rates for CALL vs. OPPORTUNISTIC invitations.

	ALL	CALL	OPPORTUNISTIC
Attended	170	113	57
DNA	47	37	10
Attendance	78%	75%	85%

Table 1 shows that the invitation rate is slower for the Opportunistic group (150 vs. 67). This is in part due to the GP being ill and away from work during part of the period. The attendance rate is higher however (85% vs 75%).

Results also indicate that substantially more appointments are changed when they have been offered to the Call group by letter. The Opportunistic group have an opportunity to choose a suitable date when the appointment is made.

This difference has an effect on the 'utilization' of the health check clinic. The 'wasted' slots arise because there is often not time to reallocate a slot when a patient rearranges an appointment. The greater number of DNAs in the Call group also reduces utilization, of course.

Patients' views on the invitation were obtained and analysed from the Post Screening questionnaire. At this stage in the study there appears to be little difference between the patients' views on the methods of invitation. For example, there was no difference between the groups in the extent to which patients expressed worry or felt under pressure to attend, and both groups were equal in their level of interest in and satisfaction with the invitation.

The one difference that did arise was that the Call group of patients reported that the appointment time was harder to make. This is consistent with the greater number of changed appointments and DNAs for the Call group.

Discussion

Although the study is not yet complete, some interesting findings are already emerging. The main ones are summarised below:

- The Opportunistic method results in a higher attendance rate to the first invitation

- However, less patients were actually invited Opportunistically, and the Call method produced more patients at the health check clinic.

- However, the Call method also produced more wasted bookings in the clinic. The Opportunistic method has higher utilization of resources.

- The Opportunistic method seems to be particularly useful for patients who are less likely to respond to an invitation. For example, non-returners of the Health Questionnaire were as likely as returners to attend for screening if they were invited Opportunistically, whereas less responded when invited by letter.

- We observed that for some patients the GPs use the Opportunistic tag in the notes to pass on patient specific information to the nurse who will carry out the screening. This facility to pass on messages linked to the patient invitation should therefore be a design requirement when we convert to Opportunistic prompting (tagging) using consulting room terminals.

- Patients who do not attend have the following characteristics:

    they perceive the major causes of premature death as less serious;

they believe their health depends less on their own actions; and they have a tendency to be more worried about what might happen during a health check.

Conclusion

What is the Best Method of Invitation?
To be definitive, we need much more data from a variety of practices. But the pattern that is emerging is that the Opportunistic method is more cost effective in use of resources and more convenient for the patients. However, it is unable to reach all patients within the timescale that is likely to be necessary. This is in part due to a substantial number of patients not visiting the surgery within the time period, but also because they may not be invited when they do visit.

From a computer simulation of consulting rates for the target population we have shown that it is possible to achieve 90% screening of female patients within 2 years provided that at least 3 out of every 4 are Opportunistically invited to a health check when they consult, but that to get the corresponding 90% of male patients will take 5 years, if left to the Opportunistic method alone. Thus it will usually be necessary to 'sweep-up' patients by the Call method if they have not been invited Opportunistically. It would also be possible, and it may be desirable, to identify in advance those patients who are unlikely to be picked up Opportunistically and to Call them from the start.

From the empirical data we are gathering in our case study practices, we will also be able to establish practice and population profiles. From these a practice will be able to assess the difficulty of achieving its targets given its own unique case-mix of patients, and its own internal organization.

References

1.'Promoting Better Health' (1987). Department of Health White Paper. London, HMSO

2.Fitter, M.J., Garber, J.R., Herzmark, G.A., Robinson, D. and Jones R.V.H. (1986). A Prescription for Change: A Report on the Longer Term Use and Development of Computers in General Practice. London: HMSO.

3.Pill, R., French, J., Harding, K., and Stott, N.C.H. (1988). Invitation to attend a health check in a general practice setting: comparison of attenders and non-attenders. Journal of the Royal College of General Practitioners, 38, 53-6.

4.Fullard, E., Fowler, G., and Gray, M. (1987). Promoting prevention in primary care: controlled trial of low technology, low cost approach. British Medical Journal, 294, 1080-2.

International Primary Care Computing
G.M. Hayes and N. Robinson (Editors)
Elsevier Science Publishers B.V. (North-Holland)
© IMIA, 1991

4.2 Opportunistic Preventive Health Care - Does it Work?

Dr R M Crampton

Computer Fellow, Royal Australian College of General Practitioners, 43 Lower Fort Street, Sydney, NSW, 2000., AUSTRALIA.

Abstract
This paper will describe a project in a group of computerised Australian General Practices in which a study will be made on practitioner recording behaviour of the effect of prompting him/her to perform preventive health care measures determined to be "overdue". The project is scheduled to commence its operational phase in April 1990.

Aim

The aim of the Computerised Opportunistic Preventive Health Care Prompting Project (COPHCPP) is to assess the effect of computer generated prompting of certain preventive health behaviours on the recording behaviour of doctors using a computerized medical records system.

The research question being investigated is:

Does computer generated prompting of certain medical practitioner behaviours, which have been identified as overdue preventive health behaviours, increase the recording of those behaviours within a computerized medical records system?

Background - CAPP (Computer Assisted Practice Project)

CAPP is a joint project between the Royal Australian College of General Practitioners and Medrecord Australia P/L which is studying the effects of the introduction of computerised medical records into Australian General Practice. CAPP is administered by the RACGP CAPP Co-ordinating Committee and co-ordinated and evaluated by the Department of Community Medicine at Monash University. CAPP is modelled on the British "Micros for GPs" Project, but, after funding was rejected by the Australian Government, it was funded partially by Medrecord P/L and partially by the participating GPs.

This Computerised Opportunistic Preventive Health Care Prompting Project forms one element of the total research study conducted under the title of the Computer Assisted Practice Project.

The CAP Project initially involved 22 practices throughout Australia - Victoria 7, NSW 7, Qld 3, WA 3, SA 2, and ran for the three years, 1986-1988. The CAP Project was extended in 1989 to involve a further 19 sites - Victoria 4, NSW 3, SA 2, WA 1, Tasmania 1, Queensland 8.

From the original CAPP sites (22), 3 have elected not to be involved in the COPHCP Project - 1 each from NSW, Victoria and Queensland. One practice from CAPP-II has also joined the project.

The demographic details of these 20 practices are:
- 11 practices 1.5 full-time equivalent (FTE), 9 practices = 2 FTE, for a total of 45 practitioners

- Victoria 6, NSW 7, Queensland 2, WA 3, SA 2

- Metropolitan 13, Provincial 5, Rural 2

Each practice in CAPP has had the Medrecord Patient Medical Records and Patient Accounting system installed. This is a multi-user PICK operating system based package designed for maintaining full clinical records plus all aspects of practice financial management on-line.

It is primarily structured in modules, which include Patient Identification, Social History, Medications, Pathology results, X-ray, Immunisations, Progress Notes, Correspondence and Recalls (reminders). Information is entered usually through a Consultation Routine, which creates a Progress Note, and allows direct updating of the other modules. All entries can be problem coded using the ICHPPC system. Information is retrieved by module or by a summary routine "Profiles", which returns either a pre-selected subset (Selected Profile, eg. Social History, last Progress Note, Current Problems and Current Medications), all information about a specific problem (Problem Profile), or all information (Full Profile). These can be displayed on screen, printed prior to the consultation (Encounter Sheet), or transferred to an integrated word processor.

CAPP-I (1986-88) studied the effects of installing a computerised medical records system on the practices involved. A report on the first 12 months was presented at Medinfo 89. The full report has recently been presented to the RACGP Council, and various papers are expected to be submitted for publication soon.

CAPP-II (which was recruited and installed in 1989 and commenced operations in 1990) is a program development project in which user feedback is intended to guide the development direction for the medical records product. The first round of data input has been received.

The COPHCP Project is a specific research project funded by the CAPP funding agreement between Medrecord and the RACGP.

Method

Preliminary Development
The "Recalls" module within the medical records system was initially designed to accept any doctor initiated recalls and subsequently produce lists or letters after the "due date" was passed. A modification to the program (the Consult Routine) caused the automatic display of these "Recalls" at each consult, and hence these recalls could then be termed to be displayed "Opportunistically".

The COPHCP project required further modifications to be made to the Medrecord Medical Records Program. These created:

i)   Preventive Health Care Schedule - a schedule of recommended preventive health care behaviours for varying groups based on age and sex - see Tables 1 and 2.

ii)   Preventive Care Prompts - to indicate those patients and those parameters who have "outstanding" preventive care according to the Preventive Health Care Schedule.

iii)A Preventive Care Programme - which searches back through each patient's medical record. For each preventive parameter for which no relevant record is found, a Preventive Care Prompt is created. These are called "System Generated" prompts as opposed to those which are input by a practitioner, but they are stored in the Recalls module and tagged to identify their origin. Appendix 1 outlines this creation process.

The flexibility to search a selected set of patients based on their record numbers has been incorporated into the programme, but the project will address the whole patient population that exists on the computer.

Each practitioner in the project uses a computer terminal in his/her consulting room for the real-time recording of clinical data. (The philosophy behind the development of these routines was that no further work should be required of the practitioner to maintain the integrity and accuracy of the prompts).

The Preventive Care Prompts are displayed on screen to the practitioner at the commencement of each consultation, and subsequently on demand throughout the consultation.

Study Method
For the purposes of the research project, these Prompts can be either displayed or suppressed by the researcher for fixed periods of time.

The 20 practices will be allocated into four groups, A1, A2, B1 and B2, in such a way as to give equal distributions of practices based on size (FTE) and location (rural/provincial/metropolitan) between "super-groups" A and B.

Over 3 consecutive two-month periods, identified as periods 1, 2 and 3, the Preventive Prompts will be displayed (ON) or suppressed (OFF) in each of the groups of practices according to the following table:

	A1	A2	B1	B2
PERIOD 1	ON	ON	OFF	OFF
PERIOD 2	OFF	OFF	ON	ON
PERIOD 3	ON	OFF	ON	OFF

Analysis

Within each practice, on-going counts will be maintained of the number and type of Prompts displayed (when ON) or suppressed (when OFF). At the conclusion of each two-month period, a retrospective count of the number of recordings of each preventive health care parameter will be taken.

Comparisons will then be made between ON and OFF periods, and conclusions about possible effects of the display of relevant Preventive Health Care Prompts on the recording behaviour of doctors will be drawn.

Numerical Analysis
The following analyses are planned:

Within each group A1 - B2, for each period I - III, a comparison will be made for each preventive parameter between the number of individual prompts displayed/suppressed versus the number of individual preventive health care parameters recorded (whether overdue or not). This comparison will form the basis of the conclusion about the effect of the display of preventive prompts on doctors' recording behaviour.

Within each group A1 - B2, a comparison will be made for each preventive parameter number between the individual preventive health care parameters recorded (whether overdue or not) between periods I and II, and between periods II and III. This comparison will help determine any latency effect there may be that persists after the status of the prompts have been changed in the practice.

Within each group A and B, a comparison will be made for each preventive parameter between the number of individual preventive health care parameters recorded (whether overdue or not) between periods I and II. This comparison will help to control for outside influences which may intermittently promote better preventive health care awareness.

Progress
This project was first conceived in 1987! Unfortunately, many programme delays resulting from inadequate resource allocations have continued to defer its starting date. At present, the operating version of the programme is being installed in the project sites, and real-time experience is being gained by each practitioner with the prompt creation and review process.

One pilot site in Western Australia first tested using the reminders in an opportunistic method over a two year period. In that time, he raised the penetration rate for tetanus immunisations and Pap smears from an initial figure of 30% of eligible patients covered to approximately 80% of eligible patients. He has been unable to lift the cover above that rate. That practice then tested the prompting routine over a four month period, alternating on a monthly cycle with the display of prompts on or off. The results of this phase of the project suggest a significant effect can be seen from the use of the preventive prompts, as a marked decrease in frequency of recording of preventive care behaviour was revealed during each period in which the prompts were suppressed.

Discussion

Expected Results
The following results would support the hypothesis that the preventive health care prompts had a positive effect on the practitioners' recording behaviour.
- The display of computer generated prompts correlates with an increase in the preventive care recording behaviour of this group of practitioners.

- The cessation of the prompts correlates with a decrease in the rate of preventive care recording behaviour.

The following result would not refute the hypothesis, but would modify the conclusion such that the overall usefulness of such prompts would be limited.
- The persistence of the prompts correlates with a decrease in the rate of preventive care recording behaviour.

Problems
Problems with results from this study are expected to come from three areas at least:
- i) System use

- the effect of using a new and otherwise untested routine
- ii) Dilution of results

- various factors about the use and operation of the system will result in an over-recording of prompts displayed and a possible under-recording of the data entered.

- The interpretations that one may place on the conclusions could be challenged on the grounds of Controls for the results and of self-selection of the practices to be involved in the project.

Conclusion

Few are possible at this stage. Most definitely, programme development is complex and difficult, and medical programme development needs the constant attention of a medical practitioner to oversee the process.

The pilot results indicate that it is worthwhile to continue with the project.

The practitioners currently using the system in trial phase are very satisfied with their use of the system, but are already suggesting and requesting modifications and improvements to the software.

I expect to be able to report the outcome of this project by the end of 1990.

Reference

1.Health Maintenance Guide, Canadian College of Family Physicians, 1983.

Acknowledgement

This research is supported by the RACGP and Medrecord Australia Pty. Ltd. through the Computer Assisted Practice Project.

Table One

Preventive Health Care Parameters

1.	Alcohol intake
2.	Blood pressure
3.	Breast examination
4.	Head circumference
5.	Measles/Mumps immunization
6.	Papanicolaou smear
7.	Serum cholesterol and triglycerides
8.	Smoking
9.	Tetanus immunization
10.	Weight

Table Two

Preventive Health Care Schedule

1. Alcohol intake	- once	- all patients	**15 yo**
2. Blood pressure	- 5 years	- all patients	**16 - 39 yo**
	- 2 years	- all patients	**40 - 74 yo**
	- once	- all patients	**74 yo**
3. Breast examination	- 1 year	- all females	**16 - 64 yo**
4. Measles/Mumps immunization			
	- once	- all patients	**15mo - 15yo**
5. Papanicolaou smear	- 1 year	- all females	**16 - 60 yo**
6. Serum cholesterol and triglycerides			
	- 5 years	- all patients	**20 yo**
7. Smoking	- once	- all patients	**15 yo**
8. Head circumference	- 1 year	- all patients	**birth-15yo**
9. Weight	- 1 year	- all patients from birth	
10. Tetanus immunization			
- Schedule 1	- all patients birth-5yo		
- 10 years	- all patients 5 yo		

Schedule 1

2 mo	4 mo	6 mo	18 mo	5 yo

Appendix 1

The ten parameters divide into 2 groups of five.

The first five, Smoking, Alcohol, BP, Weight and Head Circumference can be termed "fixed field" parameters because there are specific fields throughout the Patient Master File, Progress Notes File and Paediatric File for the recording of the information.

The second five, Breast Examination, Tetanus, Measles/Mumps, Cholesterol/Triglyceride and Pap Smear are termed "free field" because there is no specific field in the record where this information is always recorded.

A programme has been incorporated into Medical Records Release MR3.2 which searches the appropriate files for these ten parameters for each patient as far back as indicated by the Preventive Health Care Schedule (Table 2). For example, when determining the status of Blood Pressure recording for a 42 yo female, the programme searches for a Blood Pressure recording in the Progress Notes over the past 2 years.

This programme will run overnight (it takes some time!) after the backup run, and will create a Recall record (a "System Generated Recall") for each parameter for each patient.

International Primary Care Computing
G.M. Hayes and N. Robinson (Editors)
Elsevier Science Publishers B.V. (North-Holland)
© IMIA, 1991

4.3 Screening:

Report

Chairman, Bernard Richards

Dept. of Computer Science UMIST Sackville Street Manchester M60 1QD UK

Presenter, Mike Fitter

MRC/ESRC Social & Applied Psychology Unit, University of Sheffield, Sheffield S10 2TN UK

Discussant, Michael Crampton

Computer Fellow, Royal Australian College of General Practitioners, 43 Lower Fort Street, Sydney, NSW, 2000., AUSTRALIA.

Rapporteur, Angie Daniels

Oxford Community Health Project Oxford RHA Old Road Headington Oxford UK

Comments and Conclusions

The first paper discussed a project to evaluate the use of opportunistic screening using computer generated prompts and reminders versus screening by computer generated call letters.

The discussant has been involved in a project aimed at evaluating the use of computer prompts for opportunistic screening over a six month period.

It was agreed that screening should cover not only preventive care but the continuing care of the already diagnosed chronic disease patient, offering prompts and reminders to ensure good standards of care and monitoring of progress. The main benefit of the electronic medical record over the handwritten record is that the computer will inform you not only of the information that is present but, sometimes more importantly, the information that is missing. A set of rules and reminders are needed for every cohort of patients. These can then be used opportunistically or used to send out call letters.

In countries where there is no fixed patient register opportunistic screening will be more valuable than a call system and for the future there may be enormous benefits for health screening using smart card technology.

The accuracy of the patient register, especially in inner-city areas with a highly mobile population, can present enormous problems to effective screening. Attempts to meet target levels for specific screening procedures may fail unless the accuracy of the register can be improved. There is little hard evidence about the total potential uptake rate, even in a stable population, and the maximum possible uptake may prove to be well below 100%.

The computer has a very positive role to play in patient selection for screening, but the rules and protocols need to be dynamic, changing as patient profiles change and morbidity data is recorded.

The need for a terminal on every doctor's desk is more difficult to rationalise, but in the prevention of iatrogenic disease there is no substitute for the relevant information available on the doctor's desk at the time of prescribing. Encounter sheets for collecting data and providing opportunistic reminders are very useful if there is no terminal on the doctor's desk. A computer system with family linkage can also improve the uptake rate from opportunistic screening, as family members can be targeted for some non-sensitive screening invitations for their close relatives, e.g. parents for children's immunisations, spouse for partner's check-up etc. This can be particularly useful for improving uptake rates in countries with no fixed patient register.

Patient used questionnaires on the computer may be a valuable way of obtaining baseline data to enhance screening programmes and can reduce the amount of time that the doctor or nurse spends gathering routine data. In some areas patient literacy may make this impossible, but the computer can help by translating information into the patient's mother tongue.

International Primary Care Computing
G.M. Hayes and N. Robinson (Editors)
Elsevier Science Publishers B.V. (North-Holland)
© IMIA, 1991

5   MEDICAL AUDIT

Chairman, Mr Stephen Kay

Medical Informatics Group, Dept Computer Science, Manchester University, Oxford Rd , Manchester M13 9PL UK

Presenter, Dr Graham Page

Mantra Consultancy Ltd, 9 Nightingale Lane, Earlsdon,Coventry CV5 6AY UK

Discussant Dr Martin Lawrence

West Street Surgery, 12 West Street, Chipping Norton, Oxon OX7 5AA UK

Rapporteur Dr Bob Bowles

Upper Knapps Shire Lane Lyme Regis Dorset DT7 3ET UK

Introduction

The workshop was introduced by referring to Sheldon's prize winning essay on medical audit[1] back in 1982. In particular, given the nature of the meeting, it was suggested that his five steps should be examined with respect to computer support. (In the event, the more sociological and political aspects of the subject were considered more than the purely technical). The relationship and scope of the types of audit were briefly considered and how structure, process and outcome were related to patient care. The 'patient' was a source of difficulty throughout the discussion.

The following quotes, not all in context, were used to stimulate the discussion:
'The purpose of medical audit is to improve the quality of care'[2]

'useful audit as a by product of routine data capture is unrealistic'[3]

'It is much harder to audit a patient than to audit a disease'[4]

'good medical records are essential.... an approach based on standard
     case-note files or on local databases ...is manifestly bound to fail'[5]

C.D. Shaw, in the March edition of the BMJ[6] this year, described four phases of introducing Medical Audit: philosophical, organisational, practical and invasive. Two of Shaw's four phases were the topics of the discussants. The first, by Dr Page, concentrated more on the philosophical phase attempting to clarify terms and meaning. The second discussant, Dr Martin Lawrence, had moved on from the 'earlier' phases to Shaw's practical phase, concerned with the 'what' and 'how', and had implemented a scheme in his Practice.

Concluding Remarks

The discussion was lively and wide ranging. Other working sessions during the day, notably the one on coding and classification, were pertinent to the debate. It was impoverished, however, by the fact that all the participants were from the UK. Consequently, it was not possible to consider the meaning of medical audit across different cultures. The markedly different health care delivery systems, legislation, the organisation, structures, processes and measurements of outcome are all variables which may affect what is understood by the term. For example the UK NHS with the GP as 'gate keeper', possessing a unique, centralised repository of a patient's clinical data, is quite different from a more 'contact' centered organisation of healthcare as found in West Germany; the latter generates many occurrences of unlinked records and has more restrictions on the interchange of data.

The other major uncharted area which could not be satisfactorily addressed was the notion of Shared Care. This, too, was primarily because of the group's composition and, indeed, partly due to the shortage of available time to discuss such a topic. It is perhaps too convenient to regard this subject as being the exclusive concern of clinical audit rather than medical audit. The wider context may well be required to interpret the relatively local findings. Although Shaw regarded the phases of medical audit to be serial in time, it is clear that his observations were made to simplify what is in reality a complex development. Certainly, the conviction of the second speaker was that it was necessary to 'make a start' somewhere and that it was not feasible to wait until all was clarified. At the same time, the need for clarification and further definition is an on-going task which will be assisted by practical experimentation. The subject of medical audit is both controversial and confusing. The workshop reflected both aspects and posed more questions than it answered. But perhaps such a discussion and outcome are no bad things. The iterative nature of the subject's development will undoubtedly ensure a continuing debate. The value of reporting and documenting such discussions is to reduce the likelihood of the cycle degenerating into the merely circular.

References

[1] Sheldon MG. (1982/8) Medical Audit in General Practice. RCGP Occasional paper 20.

[2] Baker R. (1990) Problem solving with audit in general practice. BMJ. 300:378-80

[3] Nixon SJ. (1990) Defining essential hospital data. BMJ 300:380-1

[4] Stott NCH and Davies R. (1975) Clinical and Administrative Review in general practice. J. RCGP 25:888-896

[5] Goodyear OM. (1989) Medical Audit and Shared care. In proceedings of Information Technology and Shared Care (British Medical Informatics Society and Bull HNC)

[6] Shaw CD. (1990) Criterion Based Audit.BMJ 300:649-51

International Primary Care Computing
G.M. Hayes and N. Robinson (Editors)
Elsevier Science Publishers B.V. (North-Holland)
© IMIA, 1991

5.1   Audit

Discussion Report

It does not matter where one starts in the cycle provided one begins. It is easy to set impossible standards, but the basis is to start collecting data, review it after three months, and if necessary try again. This cycle is like that of Pluto: try, fail, try again, fail better.

There is a lot to be said for thinking about a problem, collecting data about it, and then trying to come to a conclusion, even though it is only a preliminary trial. Many studies are done this way, and a lot of so-called trials which are really hypothesis generating surveys, which are written up as trials and people put "p values" on the results.

An example would be that of an anaesthetist who jotted down a set of minimum data for obstetric audit, and was horrified to find it adopted as a national standard, since people were so anxious to get hold of anything. He was the first to admit it had not been thought through in detail.

Useful Audit

The Chairman was quoted as saying that useful audit as a by-product of routine data capture is unrealistic.

Useful audit which is not a by product of routine data capture is unrealistic. Life is not long enough to set up specific recording systems for every problem. The demands on general practice to produce information now, are so great that the only way you ever have time to think of a problem is to collect a lot of data automatically, which is how we practice clinically. During surgery we put much of our work on automatic pilot, leaving ourselves time to think about the difficult areas, and it is the same with audit.

Experience with inpatient data in hospitals which was only in the form of data sets on computer was inadequate for audit, whereas the GP remains in constant touch with his patients and has a clinical record.

Carrying Out Audit

In what way is audit carried out? If the objectives are not understood, and it is necessary to talk it through all the time, it is of little use trying to carry it out. Until terms are defined, it is like going into a shop, offering a penny when you are asked for a pound, and saying that's what a pound means to me, and expecting to get the goods. You won't.

I applaud the pragmatism of audit based on data; sooner or later you have to confront the situation. It's a bit like saying the helmsman of a sailing boat never leaves the helm - there is water coming into the boat and the helmsman bails the cockpit, despite the fact that the water is coming in from the front of the boat and he will inevitably sink if he persists in this action.

One challenge is the issue of the distinction between medical and clinical audit; another is that of starting to look at things which were not looked at previously. A major challenge is that of objective setting: who does it, and how they do it? It is not good enough to talk platitudes in terms of what we can comfortably measure already. There is good evidence that the only audits which change practices are the ones which are set up in response to the recognition of a problem.

The solution is to record a lot of data automatically; this then gives the opportunity to construct an audit on something that interests you from the mass of data already collected. Pragmatism is necessary; there must be realism and compromise. The door must not be closed to new initiatives, and the danger of putting audit into a watertight compartment must be avoided. The quality of care, outcome and resource use is important, otherwise judgments are made which have a consequence in other areas, leading to unsatisfactory results.

As an example, UK visitors to the USA when looking at hospital discharge rates, announced that the UK scenario would be different, since the UK's more highly developed primary care system and discharge planning on the day of admission would result in a shorter length of stay. When challenged about the assumption that length of stay would be less in the UK than in the American system, the home team admitted that they had not thought this assumption through.

Regarding sharing data, under the new NHS GP contract relating to purchasers and providers of services in the marketplace for hospital services, there was an assumption of access to GP collected data. The GPs felt strongly that the contract was between family doctor and patient and embraced confidentiality of data. The concept of this personal contract appeared alien to those outside the GP scene who gave the impression that they were entitled to access to personal data which had been collected by the GP.

Way back in 1970 Bob Johnson recorded as much clinical data as possible, having no idea if it would be helpful. He subsequently developed a specific type of audit, relating to symptoms and timescale. Take cough as a symptom, count time interval between recurrence of symptoms and relate it to treatment. On computer analysis, treatment with one particular drug showed a 20% recurrence rate as opposed to 10% with all other antibiotics, yet when setting up the original data collection protocols he had no idea of the outcome but had adopted a pragmatic approach.

What worries me is that audit in some way seems to be threatening. The dictionary compares it with the day of judgement. But audit may not help the outcome at all. The Establishment tends to say: perhaps we will locate this closer to the mean, or we shall analyse this in a different way; whereas it may have as much relevance to patient care or outcome as the colour of the doctor's eyes.

Others volunteered that a patient seeking treatment for tonsillitis wanted her throat treated and was not interested in having a cervical smear.

The Government's request for hospital referral rates in practice reports did not mean that they knew how to interpret them, but it was deemed to be acceptable to collect such routine data.

Collecting information is nothing to do with audit at all.

It is said that in general practice auditing the process is a good proxy to an outcome - this is dangerous. The doctor can have a sympathetic approach and the process is carried out well, but there is no affect on the outcome. We do have to get down to some rigorous outcome measurement. Patients should not be ignored in this; they have a good measure of what outcome is.

As regards medical audit, we must look at the business effort approach to the GP NHS contract in relation to targets. Also, the patient and physician between them could define targets and measure outcome. This would be transferrable across morbidity so that a whizz kid about asthma could also be measured about orthopaedics capability. This is difficult, because for a patient to die comfortably may seem to be a reasonable outcome.
It is said by GPs that for at least 50% of patients that come through the door they know what is wrong with them before they open their mouth. Also, 50% are going to get better, no matter what the GP does.

It is said also that audit is going to be the major change to affect health care. How should we maximise the potential for good? Take the instance of Training practices. If a principal wants a trainee he must go through peer audit, where two trainers from other practices come and inspect the practice. There is a parallel track of professional audit and external managerial audit.

This mixture of peer review and external pressure has been very successful. If it is left to professionals on their own, the track record is that it does not happen very well. The result is that, in general, training practices have higher standards than non training practices. Under the new contract, external independent medical advisers can help FHSAs monitor standards.

The GP scene has gone from low goals to high goals. To be accepted as a training practice, the notes have to be in chronological order - surely a minimum standard and not elitist. The expectation now is a much higher standard of record keeping for the ordinary practice.
Factual data is easy to enter, but with judgmental data current computer systems are less helpful and the doctor must be careful. A careless observer will not be transformed into a careful observer by using a computer.

Patients want of the GP accessibility and kindness. Kindness is hard to monitor, but accessibility can and should be monitored.

Patients who visit the family doctor are in general not ill - they wish to define the problem, and they are seeking reassurance. To give an example: a recent study on the treatment and outcome of otitis media showed that the effect of giving antibiotics had no effect whatsoever on outcome, and yet most mothers, if asked, want their children to have an anti-biotic. There is a danger in using this as a major criterion.

A consultants view - How do you audit the work of a hospital department? Take the work of a diagnostic department - Biochemistry. Which parameters do you use? There are departments where you could get rid of all the senior staff and probably get a better service. If the aim is to achieve structural change a different type of audit is required than if looking for output. In this type of audit it is necessary to focus more on process and on the translation from the case mix environment to the social side. An audit of that boundary would reveal how effective it is.

Satisfactory outcomes can be achieved, yet processes be poor. Similarly, good processes may not achieve satisfactory outcomes. A perfect example is a massive biochemistry machine, run by a superb small technical team for which a senior medical staff member is entirely unnecessary. The problem is that the system does some 12,000 sodium assays a week, and probably only 30 results are useful clinically. So there is a superb process within close statistical limits and quality assurance, but there is no feedback from the ward, and that is because in general lab people are bad at creating feedback loops.

The process of audit should generate feedback loops to compare processes and outcomes. It is a continuous complaint of hospital physicians that feedback is absent.
Easier access to data may mean that we are seeing the demise of a regime, and that in the new process of healthcare we will see the evolution of a technical department supplying a care team with the information it wants. We are seeing a shift in the structure of care teams. This touches on peer review amongst professionals when the outcome is the redundancy of that professional. This has been seen in the United States with the demise of the nurse practitioner because the doctor felt threatened. Do primary health care teams need the pre eminent GP? Some of these exercises are threatening.

Another example occurred in a comparison of results of home versus hospital coronary care. Before the formal presentation the hospital physicians had the results leaked that hospital treatment gave the best results, and the consultants were pleased. When told that a mistake had been made and that home treatment displayed better results, the hospital staff questioned the validity of the study.

The results of audit should be published without pressures on how the results might be interpreted or used. There should be a commitment, particularly on the part of management, to act on the basis of the outcome of the audit before it is begun.

Summary by Chairman

- Data should be collected pragmatically
- The areas where data is not collected routinely need special attention

- Audit is cyclical; one-off analysis is unscientific
- Feedback is a requirement

The chairman's remarks were rounded off by a plea from the audience for the prevention of the massaging of figures and political bias in the national and medical scene.

International Primary Care Computing
G.M. Hayes and N. Robinson (Editors)
Elsevier Science Publishers B.V. (North-Holland)
© IMIA, 1991

5.2   Audit

Rapporteur, Dr Bob Bowles

What is Audit?
The first thing I have found is that the terms medical audit, clinical audit and peer review are used by different people to mean different things and often to mean the same thing, so it is necessary first to define what we are talking about.

For the most mechanistic, the term audit is used by accountants for an independent review to ensure proper accounting procedures have been followed, and that nobody's fingers have been in the till.

The Audit Commission, with which we are likely to get more closely acquainted, is concerned only with value for money - efficiency. In 1991 they will be looking at pathology, day care services and estate management.

The Royal Colleges, including the Royal College of General Practitioners, are concerned to establish ultimate audit.

Peer review is by contrast a self-regulatory mechanism aimed at improving the quality and effectiveness of services. It can be local, and carried out within a practice or within a an area. It should involve analysis of the quality of medical care, including the procedures used for diagnosis and treatment, the use of resources and the resulting outcome and quality of life for the patient.

International Primary Care Computing
G.M. Hayes and N. Robinson (Editors)
Elsevier Science Publishers B.V. (North-Holland)
© IMIA, 1991

5.3   Audit Workshop

Presentation Dr Graham Page

Mantra Consultancy Ltd, 9 Nightingale Lane, Earlsdon,Coventry CV5 6AY UK

How is Audit Carried Out?

Just as there are different interpretations of the term audit, so there are a variety of different ways in which it is carried out.
Much traditional peer review concentrates on a review of process where the outcome is below medical expectations, e.g. enquiries into peri-natal mortality, peri-operative deaths. This removes the majority of cases where routine statistics do not give any crude indication of unfavourable mention in the use of these names:

Peer Review - should be used to refer to a process within the peer groups concerned only with the quality and standards of service. It could be internal and self-regulatory or external and concerned with accreditation or status (RRCP Fellowship).

Medical Audit - should refer to audit carried out by Doctors for whatever purpose. It should include assessment of resource use and include the effectiveness and efficiency of the whole health care team . Clinical standards of care are not excepted.
In the future medical audit will involve the setting of precise, measurable objectives related to need and covering all elements of medical care - diagnosis, treatment and outcome. I would make a plea for this not to take place in water tight compartments, but to cover the whole of hospital and outcome.

Another method, used in some hospitals and some practices, is based on the review of random selected records by a colleague. There is no comparative element in this, and the judgments on the adequacy of care remain largely subjective. A more systematic approach is offered by criterion based audit, used in
Australia and the USA. The topic chosen can be a diagnosis, an investigation, a treatment, or presenting symptom. Key areas of case management are defined.

Finally, there is audit based on fully developed and agreed protocols, setting standards and parameters, covering diagnosis, treatment and outcome and including resource use such as length of stay, appropriateness of investigations, etc. This extracted from medical records by a non-medical analyst are set for each.
Charles Shaw (Kings Fund) has suggested the following areas for in-patient care:

Referral	Treatment
History	Follow-up
Examination	Outcome
Investigation	Community care.

A stay in hospital is rarely more than one incident in a spectrum of care, and the long term outcome is seen often only in the community. By this process, I see the apparent conflict between quality and efficiency disappearing. As Donald Irvine has said:

Good patient care is the right care given to the right people in the right place at the right time.

A patient requires the right amount of care - not more, not less. Thus, high quality care is cost effective care, and the key elements in any systematic audit are clearly the patient register and clinical records.

The patient register must be up to date, accurate and accessible. It should include not only name, address, age and sex, but date of registration with the practice. Retrospective audit may need to exclude those who have just registered and include those who have just left.

The medical record needs to be comprehensive but concise, accessible and capable of being sorted on a number of parameters. A computerised summary with an agreed content and level of detail is the obvious answer. There are systems to do this, some already do this, but for those about to start the amount of work required to set it up and maintain it is not to be underestimated.

The prospect of sharing information between hospital and primary care for audit purposes raises many issues, both ethical and technical. But the problems should not deter anyone from starting audit or peer review. It should be based initially on sharing information about cost effectiveness and encompass both quality and efficiency.

Conclusion

I have said nothing so far about information or computing. My aim has been to provide a background for debate, setting out the issues rather than bringing solutions.

During the presentation the speaker, Dr Graham Page, was challenged about the pulling of allegedly random case notes. It was suggested that a number of case notes were rejected, often because the notes were incomplete, thus tending to a biased sample.

Presentation

Stephen Kay

I started off by doing a presentation of my own and quoted Sheldon with the five steps of medical audit.

The reason for starting it like that was to stimulate the group to discuss the informatics side. That was the last thing we did on informatics. We realised that the two words MEDICAL and INFORMATICS are very difficult and that, like medical audit, they could be seen as two ideas that are unhappy bed fellows.

Information and medical practice do not seem to fit; nor does medical practice and audit. There seems to be an unlikely meeting of minds. We realised that medical audit was not only a technical problem, but there was a sociological and political component as well. We spent much time talking about medical problems, the threats, the problems, and the worries - and we occasionally mentioned a computer and how it got in the way.

In primary care anyway the collection of routine data is the starting point; there is no need to do anything special. There may be other issues and problems that have arisen that need addressing, and in those cases there will be need for a special type of audit.

Audit should be cyclic. There is no reason for one-off; the scientific process demands that results can be repeated, and to achieve value for money it would need to be repeated over a course of time; readjust, get feedback and move on. It was important that medical audit was not done in a vacuum; it had to affect practice.

We were conscious of the shortage of time and that issues such as shared care had not been tackled.

Prof David Metcalf, introducing a BMJ article, compared audit with a searching examination - a day of judgement. Accuracy is important - Audit in the White paper is not only about medical audit, whatever that means, but also about the audit of data, and its quality. As regards routine collection, one has to have the means to collect good data at the time and use it properly.

Tactics in Zulu wars sidetracked us.

International Primary Care Computing
G.M. Hayes and N. Robinson (Editors)
Elsevier Science Publishers B.V. (North-Holland)
© IMIA, 1991

6 COMMUNICATIONS
Chairman's Report

Professor Paul Grob

Robens Institute, University of Surrey, Guildford, UK

Introduction
It can be argued that electronic data transfer will be the growth area in the next decade. During the past few years, we have seen enormous advances in stand-alone computing. I think the next growth area will be into the field of networking with all the inherent advantages and risks.

In a European context, there is a huge effort to create a Common Market of information exchange. This is both at a technical level so that satellites and 'phones can talk to each other, but also at a personal level so that individuals in this field can also communicate with each other. This involves the agreeing of common protocols, taxonomies and nomenclatures. The difficulties of European standardisation have been expressed elegantly by the phrase "the nice thing about European standards is that there are so many of them to choose from"! The EEC-funded projects RACE, AIM, DELTA, all have been designed to create this harmony of information exchange. The development of integrated systems development networks (ISDN) will allow huge changes in the field of broadband communication.

In the United Kingdom the changes within the National Health Service in such areas as audit or budget holding now make it obligatory that satisfactory information exchange systems are developed and implemented. The piecemeal development in the past must be regarded as no longer satisfactory. We cannot continue to allow ourselves to lose the opportunities that the Health Service has created to provide common standards and common systems in the field of computing.

International Primary Care Computing
G.M. Hayes and N. Robinson (Editors)
Elsevier Science Publishers B.V. (North-Holland)
© IMIA, 1991

6.1 Patient Held Record in Health Care Communications

Dr D. Markwell,

93 Wantage Road Reading Berks. UK

Introduction

Communication of clinical information within health services is required for good management, individual patient care and research. There is overlap between these requirements but each has its own characteristics and offers its own opportunities. This paper considers the role of records carried by the patient as part of a strategy for patient oriented electronic communication.

Over the past few years experiments with computer readable patient held records have taken place in several countries including the United Kingdom. The question I wish to address is, "do computer readable patient held records fit into health care communication strategy?". To attempt to answer this question I will first deal briefly with a number of other questions.

- Are patient held records of value?

- Do computer readable cards offer benefits?

- How do cards relate to other methods of electronic communications?

- Does a suitable technology exist?

- What do we know from past and present trials?

- How should patient cards be implemented?

Are patient held records of value?

Patient held medical records are not new. A prescription taken by a patient to a pharmacy is a patient held record. Diabetic and antenatal cooperation cards, carried by patients hold a written subset of the medical record appropriate to the particular condition. Steroid, anticoagulant, blood group and allergy warning cards, Medic-alert jewellery, the European health card and discharge notes given to a patient leaving hospital are also examples of written patient held records.

Unlike any other means of communication the patient is always present when he needs medical intervention. History suggests that the patient has been a useful transporter of his own paper based clinical data for many years.

Do computer readable cards offer benefits?

The advantages of computer readable patient held records include durability, size, information capacity, legibility, multilingual functions, reduction of double entry and avoidance of inconsistencies caused by transcription errors. If a single credit card sized piece of plastic can fulfil the role of dozens of pieces of paper we might expect this to be easier to carry and of more recognisable importance. With a higher carrier rate the efficiency of patient carried communication will improve.

How do cards relate to other methods of electronic communications?
Patient held records are not a replacement for other methods of electronic communication of patient records. They are however an important component in providing communication facilities appropriate to the individual patient. The available methods of electronic communication can be divided into three complementary groups according to whether the sender, receiver or subject controls the communication. Electronic mail is sender controlled, database interrogation is receiver controlled and patient held records are subject controlled.

Electronic mail transfers responsibility for acting on the contents of the message from its sender to the person to whom it is addressed. For referrals from one professional to another, for reports or results, administrative returns and aggregation of research data it has many advantages over a patient held record. However it cannot efficiently handle the transfer of information between professionals where there is no formal referral or ensure that data about each patient is available when and where it is needed. This would require that the person holding the information was aware of all the future information needs of the patient.

Remote interrogation of another system is of value for strictly controllable applications where a particular user has access to a limited subset of patient records. However to provide clinical information for each patient when and where it is needed requires more than 100,000 access points in the UK from which authorised persons would be able to interrogate the records of any patient. Security measures and indeed the system itself would be enormously expensive and with thousands of authorised users security would be hard to apply effectively.

A patient held record contains information from one or more originators but unlike electronic mail does not define a destination. The originator takes responsibility for the decision to record information and may define the groups of people to whom it is accessible. However the patient controls when, where and by whom the record is readable. Even with hundreds of thousands of access points with suitable card readers a patient held record is not accessible without the physical presence of the card. Security mechanisms such as use of a PIN, password or encryption reduce the risks if the patient held record is lost but the primary security mechanism is the patient.

The appropriate uses of patient held records
Patient held records are not suitable for messages which must precede the patient such as a referral request which must reach a consultant before an appointment is made. Electronic mail controlled by the sender is more appropriate for this. However a patient held record may usefully communicate events occurring after the referral and before the appointment.

Patient held records are not suitable for messages which must follow the patient such as the delivery of a laboratory result available hours after a sample is taken. Electronic mail from the laboratory or controlled remote system interrogation by the doctor are more appropriate for this.

The patient held record is of value whenever a patient is seen by a health professional whom he has not seen before or who for any reason does not have access to the patient's medical history. More than fifty percent of all patient encounters with health professionals occur without access to the medical record and many of these are in situations where electronic mail or on line access would be impossible or unhelpful.

The patient can make his patient held record available to dentists, opticians and pharmacists whom he consults without formal referral. It can allow a doctor to access and update a patient record in the patient's home or during unscheduled encounters. It can be read by doctors on call from other practices or deputising agencies. While away from home or when moving to a new locality a patient held record can facilitate continuity of care. In the case of accidents and emergencies a patient held record may be the only source of relevant medical information.

Administrative and research gains

This paper is predominantly concerned with benefits to the patient but the patient held record has other advantages. Reduction of the delays in locating patient records produces administrative economies. Continuity of records between different episodes, departments and institutions allows more accurate audit. Research benefits from a common record which follows a patient moving to a new locality. Patient held records can allow patients more freedom of choice as to whom they consult, while limiting the administrative problems of transferring the clinical record from one doctor to another.

Does the technology exist?

The simple answer is yes. Perhaps unfortunately the answer is that several potential technologies exist for computer readable cards. The choices of media range from magnetic stripe cards through memory cards, and smart cards to optical cards.

The small capacity of magnetic stripes prevents these from being used for meaningful clinical records. However as a health card identifying a patient record from a fixed database the magnetic stripe has a significant potential.

The large capacity of optical cards is offset by security considerations and the cost, size, weight and power requirements of optical card reader/writers. For the medium term future these preclude the use of optical system in hand-held or portable terminals. Despite this their high capacity suggests they may have uses for image storage and other memory intensive applications.

Cards containing simple IC memory lack security, are relatively expensive and do not comply with ISO credit card dimension and flexibility requirements of simple memory cards but currently have specialised applications in community nursing where the patient keeps the card in their home.

Smart cards combine IC memory (currently up to 8 Kbytes) and a processor. They can be mass produced cheaply and have a high level of inherent security. They can be read by cheap, small, rugged, reliable readers and have a lead in terms of the extent of previous usage. A low cost smart card reader can be built in to a hand held computer allowing the card to be read and written during domiciliary consultations or at the scene of an accident.

What do we know from past and present trials?
Worldwide there have been a large number of trials and one or two large scale implementations of computer readable patient cards. The populations covered have varied from less than a hundred up to a million and a current implementation in Spain plans to cover the full 40 million population. Generally speaking the larger systems are using the cards for identification only. One of the largest schemes storing clinical data began recently in Italy and currently involves 40,000 patients.

In the UK the evaluation of the Exeter Care Card project is currently being prepared. This project involved 2 Kbyte smart cards issued to over 8,000 patients containing up to 100 clinical entries on each card. Two hospitals, two general practices (total of eight GPs), eight pharmacies and a dentist had card read or read/write facilities.

Patient views
Since so much depends on the compliance of the patient, the views of patients involved in trials are important. In most of the trials so far patients have expressed enthusiasm and card carrying rates over 80% indicate that people take seriously the benefits even in trials which have been too small to realise the full potential of patient held records. In Exmouth, of over 8,000 cards issued, only one was returned because the patient was opposed to the idea of a patient held record.

Health professionals' views
The response of health professionals varies according to three factors:
- Their perception of the short term benefits for themselves and their patients.
- The proportion of the patients they see who have cards
- The level of integration between the card and an application which meets their other information requirements.

In general cards are well accepted by the full range of health professionals and secretarial staff who use them.

Implementation of data cards

Data Content

The data content of current computer readable patient held records varies widely. In Spain magnetic stripe cards with minimal data content have been used to identify records on a larger computer database. In both Rhydfelin, Wales and Bohulsan, Sweden, computer readable cards have been used as prescriptions. In West London optical cards are being used to replace the written maternity cooperation card. In France the Transvie system uses a smart card as a blood transfusion record.

A number of schemes have been more generalised. Such schemes include, in France, Biocarte and the Santal system, in Belgium a study instigated by the University of Louvain and in the U.K. the Exeter Care Card project. Similar projects in Italy, Austria, U.S.A, Canada, Switzerland and Japan are also under way.

Among the more generalised systems a large degree of commonality of data content has emerged. Identification and demographic information together with emergency medical data such as chronic diseases, allergies, medication and operations form the core of all these systems. The differences between systems are in the method of storage, the extent and detail of information, the media and the degree of integration with other systems.

Data structure

Information may be stored on a patient held record as free text, coded entries or a combination of both. Codes such as ICD9.CM or the compatible but more flexible Read Codes, allow more compact and precise storage of data than free text. Codes also open the possibility of cross translation allowing cards to be read and written in different languages. Free text can be read by cheaper smaller readers without the memory capacity for dictionaries needed to translate the codes but this advantage is diminishing.

The records may be of general form or there may be structured records holding pre-defined data elements. The record may be compacted or encrypted and typically each note includes the date and an authentication code of the person adding the record.

Integration with other systems

Most of the early experiments used patient held records as stand-alone miniature databases written to and read by simple application software. More recent work has integrated data on patient held records with that held on computer databases in hospitals, practices and pharmacies. In its simplest form this integration takes the form of a master database from which each card is written or updated.

In the Exeter Care Card project the patient held record is fully integrated with the AAH-Meditel GP system, the Abies hospital system and a purpose written pharmacy system. This allows the card to act as an ITURN (individually transported unpredictably routed network) rather than simply a computer readable medium.

Stand alone card systems have a limited life expectancy and have been successful only in environments without other IT applications. Any card system which is to be widely implemented must allow full integration with other applications. This requires an interface open to use by all present and future clinical and health care information systems.

Patient held records should be implemented in ways which maximise their ability to supplement other methods of communication. In particular the need for low cost hand held readers for use in the home and at other sites remote from network links must be taken into account.

The potential of computerised patient held records can only be fully realised if data originating from one system is readable by heterogeneous systems. A single hardware/software standard for patient held records is not possible while different media are used to meet different requirements.

However a generalised software interface can be defined which would allow different clinical information systems to access and interpret the data on a patient held record given hardware appropriate to the storage medium. Such a definition needs to include a translation layer making presenting the data from the card to each application using the coding system recognised by the application. Work by national and international standards bodies and the European AIM initiatives are complementing the efforts of card suppliers to move towards such a standard.

Conclusions

Written patient held records have been found useful in clinical practice over many years but have not replaced other means of communication. An effective strategy for the use of computer readable patient held records must recognise both their strengths and weaknesses.

Combining the use of sender originated electronic mail with patient held records gives those with a need to know a patient's record easy access to it while others are denied access. When a referral is made to another doctor electronic mail is the method of choice. When for any reason there is no formal referral or where a referral contains limited information patient held records provide a secure low cost means of communication which is welcomed by patients.

The main challenge is to adopt a set of guide-lines nationally and/or internationally which will allow patient held records to be made compatible with one another and used more effectively. This is a challenge which must be met for all methods of clinical information communication.

International Primary Care Computing
G.M. Hayes and N. Robinson (Editors)
Elsevier Science Publishers B.V. (North-Holland)
© IMIA, 1991

6.2 The OSI Demonstrator - An Update

Adrian V.Stokes, OBE

Principal Consultant, NHS Information Management Centre, 19 Calthorpe Road, Birmingham B15 1RP

Introduction

A previous paper discussed the background to the National Health Service OSI Demonstrator at Northampton Health Authority. This is briefly outlined in the next section. This paper is an update to the previous one and indicates progress to date, together with the work that is proposed to be carried out between now and the end of the project.

Background

In 1986, the Central OSI team (COSIT) was set up at the NHS Centre for Information Technology (now the Information Management Centre [IMC]) to facilitate the introduction into the NHS international standards in the field of 'Open systems interconnection' (OSI) - that is, the interconnection of different computer systems.

As part of its role, COSIT undertook a number of strategic studies and the results of these studies were published to the Service. In addition, it set up an in-house network at IMC (POSINET) for the purpose of obtaining first-hand experience of OSI standards and to provide a test-bed for the evaluation of OSI products. At present, POSINET implements a number of OSI standards, notably X.25 (WAN), ISO 8802-3 (CSMA/CD LAN), ISO 8571 (file transfer, access and management) and X.400 (message handling systems) and it is intended to procure an implementation of X.500 (directory services) in the near future.

In mid-1987 it was decided to demonstrate the use of OSI in a live healthcare environment and a number of health authorities were investigated. Two of these were short-listed and "opportunity studies" were undertaken in them, one funded by the Department of Trade and Industry (DTI) and the other by IMC. The results of these studies were put to the COSIT board in December 1987 and it was decided that Northampton HA should be the Demonstrator site. An application was made to the DTI for funding under their OSI awareness programme and, after a delay of nearly 11 months while the DTI re-examined their programmes, the formal Demonstrator started in November 1988.

The timescale for the Demonstrator was set for three years, the first two being intended for implementation and the third for demonstrations. Thus approximately three-quarters of the implementation phase has elapsed at the time of writing.
The timing for the Demonstrator was particularly opportune in view of the European Community Decision [2] making it mandatory to specify OSI (and other international

standards) in most public-sector procurements and in view of the NHS White Paper, [3] the implications of which are briefly discussed below.

Current Status and Development of the Demonstrator

Due to the start of the Demonstrator being delayed by some seven months from that originally planned, the implementation plans had to be revised, particularly due to the overlap of project years with financial years (in the original plans, the project was to have started in April 1988 so that the years coincided). Thus all the purchases required in the first project year needed to be fitted into the financial year i.e. the first five months of the project.

Changes to the Project

As the project progressed, various changes needed to be made as a result of experience and of the changing environment (both within Northampton HA and within the wider Health Service).

The original plans envisaged the interconnection of a number of computer systems already present in the authority by means of an X.25 wide area network (WAN) and using X.400 message handling systems ('electronic mail') for the transmission of data between the interconnected systems. Specifically, the systems to be interconnected were as follows:

> the ICL PAS (to be upgraded from a 2958 to a 2966)
>
> the Pathology PDP-11s (via a MicroVAX)
>
> a GP system (on Olivetti micros)
>
> the Accident and Emergency Clan machine
>
> Finance (using Apricots)
>
> the CUBIT Management Information System (on ICL)

The first significant change was in the GP practice. The twin Olivetti system (M-24 and M-28 connected via a BOS/LAN) was replaced by an Intel-386. The suppliers (VAMP) also provided another Intel-386 as a front-end processor in order to separate the communications from the practice processing.

Secondly, it was decided to upgrade the ICL 2966 (which had been upgraded from a 2958 as part of the Demonstrator) to a Series/39 Level 55 in preparation for a likely increase in demand and to reduce running costs. This upgrade was finally achieved in early 1990.

Thirdly, the CUBIT database system was replaced by the Walker International Ledger system running on an IBM machine at the Region. It was also decided not to include the finance department Apricot systems in the Demonstrator but instead to include an 'Arix' system running WIMS-2 for Estates. Capital asset data is transferred from this machine to the Region. An interesting problem arose during the implementation of the Demonstrator. Since it provided a suitable infrastructure for information transfer between machines, there was considerable interest in connecting other systems to the network. It was decided in principle to allow a relatively limited number of other systems to be connected, in parallel with the Demonstrator (but not formally part of it) and the first such machine to be connected was a DRS-500 for surgical audit. This was relatively straight-forward since, although the machine has a different architecture from the DRS-400 (Clan-4) used for Accident and Emergency, it has the same operating system (Unix) and hence the same software can be used.

Thus the changes to the original project are relatively small and have enhanced the usefulness of the project. The interconnected systems are:

the Patient Administration System (ICL 3955)

the Pathology PDP-11s (via a MicroVAX)

a GP system (on an Intel-386)

The Accident and Emergency DRS-400 machine

the WIMS-2 system (on Arix)

The Surgical Audit System (on DRS-500)

Current status

The project is basically on schedule - although there have been changes as the project has proceeded, including rescheduling of various activities, it is anticipated that it will be completed on time and within budget.

At the time of writing, the position is that all the hardware has been purchased and installed. The X.25 network has been installed and is fully operational; all computers used in the Demonstrator have been connected to it and are able to communicate. X.400 software has been installed on some of the computers and data has been exchanged between some of the systems. The first X.400 transmission took place at the end of 1989 between the Accident and Emergency DRS-400 and the GP Intel-386. There is also regular contact between the Demonstrator project and the POSINET system at IMC, using X.400 via BT's Packet SwitchStream (PSS).

Lessons Learnt

Clearly implementation of the Demonstrator has not been straightforward, but most of the problems have been overcome. They can be broken down into two categories, technical and managerial. This section outlines some of these problems. As the project has progressed, a daily diary has been kept of the progress and problems encountered (and, where appropriate, their solutions). At the end of the project, a detailed description will be published.

In view of the innovative nature of the project, it was expected that there would be a significant number of technical problems and these were indeed encountered. Perhaps the most significant was that of compatibility between the various systems. Although the NHS has adopted the Government OSI Profile (GOSIP4) as its functional profile and the project required all systems to conform to that profile, there were still problems of compatibility, some of which took considerable time to resolve. A particular problem area was that of addressing and routing (especially X.400 MTA routing) and, at the time of writing, not all these problems had been resolved.

Various hardware problems were also encountered. Perhaps the most significant was that a MicroVAX was ordered but a VAXserver was delivered instead. Since these look similar, it took some time to detect the error (which was, of course, immediately rectified). Considerable time was also spent in sorting out wiring problems (eg, noisy lines) but these were straightforward, although tedious.

On a more positive note, it was decided to purchase the Net-Tel X.400/X.25 software for the GP practice. Because of the considerable amount of monitoring and error detection built into the software, this system was used to detect errors in other implementations and proved a most valuable tool.

The main managerial problems encountered involved being able to contact the right people in a company at the right time. It would be advisable if, in future, any large companies taking part in such a project appointed a specific project manager who was part of the normal management structure and who had access to experts within the company. Also, the number of people in each company with the relevant expertise is very small - one or two - and such people are inevitably booked up for months ahead. Careful scheduling is therefore required, especially where it is necessary to co-ordinate between a number of companies (for example, when agreeing the MTA routing plan).

OSI and the White Paper

The NHS White Paper 'Caring for Patients' was published in early 1989. One of the clear implications of the White Paper is the need for transmission of considerably larger amounts of data than at present, especially between authorities and between hospitals and the family practitioner service. Not only is the EC Decision likely to enforce the use of OSI (depending on the value of any procurement - there is a derogation to the Decision for procurements under 100 000 ecu), but also OSI provides the only practical way to achieve such interchange efficiently and effectively.

The Demonstrator is very appositely timed, since it clearly demonstrates that the use of OSI protocols is not only the best theoretical solution but that they can be applied effectively in practice. Between now and the end of the project, there will be a large number of demonstrations, exhibitions and seminars to convey this message to as wide an audience as possible and to try to disseminate the expertise gained.

Future Plans

At present, the highest priority is to ensure that all the Demonstrator systems are able to communicate using the relevant protocols. Once this has been achieved, the information required to be transmitted will be extracted from the various systems and, on reception, stored in the appropriate place in the destination system. This work is already in progress and, for example, a discharge letter from A&E has been agreed and implemented. These letters form the 'body part' of X.400 messages being transmitted.

Once the main objectives of the Demonstrator have been achieved, there are various other items of work under consideration. Essentially, the Demonstrator will provide a suitable infrastructure for other projects. Clearly it is in the district's interests for other systems to be connected together in a similar manner. There is an appreciable cost involved in doing so, because of the hardware and software required, but once this has been achieved, there will be a fully integrated hospital and district system (cf the HISS initiative).

It was recently announced that Northampton HA would be one of the Resource Management project sites. The work already done on the Demonstrator provides a sound basis for this implementation and, of course, the operational requirement for resource management requires full OSI conformance.

Another project that is under active consideration is to use the district as the test bed for examining various proposals for the encoding of information to be transferred (eg, MEDIX).

Finally, as more OSI protocols become stable, it might be appropriate for a small number of pilot projects to be initiated to examine their utility within the healthcare context.

Summary and Conclusions

The OSI Demonstrator is a major project well on the way to completion. Despite many problems - some anticipated, others not - the project is likely to be completed on time and within budget. The use of OSI within the Health Service is likely to expand greatly in the near future, particularly in the light of the White Paper, and the experiences in Northampton HA will be invaluable in the wider implementation of OSI in the Service.

Acknowledgements

I would like to thank the members of the Project Team, especially Keith Oswin (project leader), for their work on the Demonstrator and their assistance in preparing this paper.

References

1. Stokes AV. The National Health Service OSI Demonstrator. In:L Roberts J, ed. Current perspectives in health computing 1989. Weybridge: BJHC, 1989: 7-8.

2. Stokes AV. Council Decision of 22 December 1986 on standardization in the field of information technology and telecommunications (87/95/EEC). Official Journal of the European Communities 1987; L36: 31.

3. Stokes AV. Working for Patients, CM555. London: HMSO, 1989.

4. UK Government OSI Profile (Version 3). Central Computer and Telecommunications Agency, January 1988.

Relevant international standards

X.25 (1984) Interface between data terminal equipment (DTE) and data circuit-terminating equipment (DCE) for terminals operating in the packet mode and connected to public data networks by dedicated circuit

X.400 (1984) Message Handling Systems: System Model - Service Elements

X.401 (1984) Message Handling Systems: basic service elements and optional user facilities

X.408 (1984) Message Handling Systems: encoded information type conversion rules

X.409 (1984) Message Handling Systems: Presentation transfer syntax and notation

X.410 (1984) Message Handling Systems: remote operations and reliable transfer server

X.411 (1984) Message Handling Systems: Message Transfer Layer

X.420 (1984) Message Handling Systems: interpersonal messaging User Agent Layer

X.430 (1984) Message Handling Systems: Access protocol for Teletex terminals

X.25 (1988) Interface between data terminal equipment (DTE) and data circuit-terminating equipment (DCE) for terminals operating in the packet mode and connected to public data networks by dedicated circuit

X.400 (1988) Message Handling: system and service overview

X.402 (1988) Message Handling Systems: Overall architecture

X.403 (1988) Message Handling Systems: Conformance testing

X.407 (1988) Message Handling Systems: Abstract service definition conventions

X.408 (1988) Message Handling Systems: encoded information type conversion rules

X.411 (1988) Message Handling Systems: message transfer system: Abstract service definition and procedures

X.413 (1988) Message Handling Systems: Message store: Abstract service definition

X.419 (1988) Message Handling Systems: Protocol specifications

X.420 (1988) Message Handling Systems: Interpersonal messaging system

X.500 (1988) Open Systems Interconnection - The Directory - Overview of
concepts, models and services

X.501 (1988) Open Systems Interconnection - The Directory - Models
X.509 (1988) The Directory - Authentication framework

X.511 (1988) The Directory - Abstract service definition

X.518 (1988) The Directory - Procedures for distributed operation

X.519 (1988) The Directory - Protocol specifications

X.520 (1988) The Directory - Selected attribute types

X.521 (1988) The Directory - Selected object classes

ISO 8571 File Transfer, Access and Management

Part 1: General Description

Part 2: Virtual filestore definition

Part 3: File Service Definition

Part 4: File Protocol Specification

Part 5: Protocol Implementation Conformance Statement proforma

ISO 8802 Local Area Networks

Part 3: CSMA/CD Access Method and Physical Layer specifications

International Primary Care Computing
G.M. Hayes and N. Robinson (Editors)
Elsevier Science Publishers B.V. (North-Holland)
© IMIA, 1991

7.   THIRD WORLD IT (WORKSHOP 7)

Chairman :Prof. Z. Ibrahim, Institute of Child Health Great Ormond Street London UK

Presenter :Dr Otto Reinhoff, Institute of Medical Informatics Phillips Universtat FB Humanmedizin und Klinikum Bunsenstrasse 3, D-3550 Marburg West Germany

Discussant: Dr R. Brittian, North Warwickshire Health Authority Heath End Road Nuneaton UK

Discussant: Mr R. Fawdry, Milton Keynes Hospital Milton Keynes Bucks.   UK

Rapporteur: Ms Grizelda Moules, Raspberry Cottage 87 Corsham Road Whitley Melksham Wilts. SN12 8QF UK

CHAIRMAN'S INTRODUCTION

What has science achieved for mankind if the basic necessities for the people are missing?

The "Third World" represents 80% of humanity. Science has a social responsibility to these people. However it must be realised that Third World countries are not all the same. Since the 1960's these countries have moved in different directions. Asia, which with countries of the Pacific Basin includes China,(representing one fifth of humanity,) and India together are becoming self sufficient. The countries of Latin America face large national debts and a mixture of the very rich and very poor, and the poverty of sub-Saharan Africa with contrasts with the political corruption of South Africa.

- Who controls the technology?

Competing power groups in a developing country include the urban elite, and ruling power groups, including party, military and commercial interests. Do those who control deploy the technology? or have the power to control thought processes, e.g. through newspapers and books.

- IT and the distribution of power

The use of IT must be democratised by making it cheap and easily available. Low cost ruggedised equipment with power supplies which can use solar or wind power can bring IT benefits to any rural location.

- Social control of IT

There must be a free and unbiased flow of information. Academic centres and international organisations such as WHO and UNESCO need to be involved.

- IT and a marriage of technologies

Technologies such as telephones, computers, modems and satellites links will allow use of remote data bases for agriculture, health and education. The use of video and computers in academic medical centres will make better application of existing technologies

possible, e.g. CAT scan.
- IT and decision making process.

At central level in a fast-moving world, day to day adjustments are needed. Forecasting, monitoring trends and evaluation are needed.
At a peripheral or district level, reliable data are required
instead of guess-work. This is especially important where local expertise is not available. A quick response from a centre for solutions to problems is required as well as a quick response for assessment of the size of a problem.

DR OTTO REINHOFF'S PRESENTATION FOLLOWED.
(No text was provided for inclusion in these proceedings)

FIRST DISCUSSANT
Roger Brittain
Why IT, why do we need information? Information is a response to a cascade of complexities. As the biomass is growing, so is the scale of change. Information is needed when scale increases. Natural evolution is beginning to produce artificial evolution as the brain is causing things to change. Technology is needed to do good and used to do evil. There are emotional influences and expectations.

WHO is a global information system. The charities need to get together to investigate what IT needs are so that existing computers are being put to the best use. Keyboards eg for pictograms for Chinese. There is a racism of language elitism against countries using pictograms, with the implication that they are less worthy as they missed out in inventing a phonetic alphabet. Turing machines may give an artificial test for AI, such as TRUDIE, MICKEY and SOPHIE, where information may be entered and advice given which could scare the patient. If it is powerful enough to do that, what are we involving ourselves in?

Regarding IT in the world. We need to refer to specific problems
in specific areas, and the need to bear in mind the problems of corruption and data protection which have a major role in information, IT , implementation, success or failure , use etc. The cost of information verses the cost of no information needs to be considered, the cost of knowing versus the cost of not knowing. Political control is exercised by countries. Need to distinguish between information / information technology / communication technology and data / information / knowledge. Information in USSR caused change, rather than IT which enabled it. We are now going through a knowledge revolution as we have gone through an industrial revolution. Data, knowledge and belief need to be distinguished. The growth of mental technology has been minuscule compared with the physical technology itself. (Here Geoffrey Dove voiced his disagreement with this premise.)

Brittain felt that we should not rush into buying technology before considering what we are doing and the implications for our spiritual environment. Mental technology is needed to control physical technology. Decision support is essential.

International Primary Care Computing
G.M. Hayes and N. Robinson (Editors)
Elsevier Science Publishers B.V. (North-Holland)
© IMIA, 1991

7.1 THIRD WORLD IT

The Creation Revolution and Information in the Third World (An Inquiry into the Health of Nations)

Dr Roger Brittain, Associate Professor of Community Medicine

Stewart McMorran, Chief Researcher

Expert Systems and Decision Support Unit, University of Warwick, U.K.

Introduction

This paper records issues raised in the International Medical Informatics Association (IMIA) Working Group on Information Technology for Primary Care in the Third World. Many of the issues have implications which are so broad as to make them applicable globally; the issues have consequences which are so profound that they could not be dealt with adequately in the amount of time which could be accorded in the session or the amount of space which can be afforded in a collection of proceedings. We apologise for mistakes or inadequacies which have crept in as a result of these constraints. This paper's references should be seen as an extension of the content of the Working Group.

The first issue dealt with by the Working Group was part of the group's title, "The Third World." It was unanimously agreed that the use of this concept is both historically incorrect and also misleading to the extent of being counter productive. This point has already been made many times. The Club of Rome stressed the need to break down any geographically global analyses as appropriate to the nature of the problem under discussion.

We agree with Marsden Blois that there is a need for a statement of principles, a theoretical foundation, and a conceptual structure and model for the introduction of information technology into health care. Most of the needs have been addressed exhaustively and repeatedly in humanity's long history of attempting to develop principles, theoretical foundations and conceptual structures and modelers for human knowledge belief. We shall use the word "Principia" to refer to these issues as a totality and the word "Credo" to refer to the moral, ethical, and belief structure which emerges. There is an important precedent for the explicit statement of the principles, ethics, and beliefs of health care in the Hippocratic Oath and its modern update, the World Health Organisation Oath.

The Principia is a partial attempt to begin to produce the sort of credo which must have been Marsden Blois' Holy Grail. In what follows, we shall attempt to cover, however inadequately, some of the issues involved.

A Brief History of Recording Knowledge-Belief

The amount of knowledge-belief in the world is increasing so rapidly that mankind can not use it to its full. Even so, the rate of increase is not so great as it could be since much knowledge-belief is not recorded.

There are many reasons for not recording it; among them are inadequate time, encouragement, and technology to record the individual's knowledge-belief and expertise. Usually the knowledge-beliefs - experience, expertise, and wisdom - of each unique person dies with her or him.

Knowledge-belief is obtained by the individual from the genes and by learning but what is learned is only a small part of what was and is known in the world i.e. the totality over time, space, energy and organisation of world knowledge-belief. Some of what is learned is forgotten by the individual and even that which is remembered is not always used on each occasion on which it might be of use.

For about four billion years on earth, living things have struggled to record and pass knowledge-belief from generation to generation. This paper concentrates on non-genetic (i.e. artificial) knowledge-beliefs of humans.

At first the artificial passing of knowledge-belief was done by imitation, demonstration, verbal tradition and ballads. The invention of writing enabled the earliest Egyptians, Chinese, and Mesopotamians to record knowledge-belief, and to keep these records on tablets of stone, and clay, as well as papyrus. These early records were only fragments of all that was believed and known. The library of Alexandria in Egypt contained many knowledge-beliefs of the time but was destroyed, most likely because of differences in belief between religious groups.

Eventually some advanced thinkers attempted to record much of the knowledge-belief of their day i.e. to create encyclopedias. For well over two thousand years, attempts to create encyclopedias have been limited by the technology of their period.

Limitations included the fact that knowledge-belief had to be recorded on and locked to paper or its equivalent and its content was what, to conventional minds, was expressible in written prose and notation, e.g. for music and mathematics. The human mind is capable of expert interactive, N-dimensional knowledge-belief manipulation. Paper limited the recording of what went on in the brain, to two dimensions and writing limited it to a one dimensional, static, linear representation on that paper.

The Creation Revolution

Humanity is involved in a revolution in its own creativity and evolution; the brain itself is influencing its own evolution. At least three major revolutions are currently taking place.

The industrial revolution began in the 19th century and continues to provide machines and tools which extend our physical ability (Bell, D. (1974)). It also brought with it what some sages predicted would be a destruction revolution (Beccaria, D. (1763), Malthus, R. (1798)). Some still predict this (Forrester, J. (1971), Meadows, D. (1970), United Nations Intergovernmental Panel on Climatic Change (1990)).

The knowledge-belief revolution began in the 20th century (Bell, D. (1974), Handy, C. (1984)) and provides the tools of advanced information technology which extend our mental ability.

These two revolutions are culminating in a third, a revolution in human creativity which takes advantage of all the products of the industrial and knowledge-belief revolutions. Some of the tools of this creation revolution include belief networks (BN), expert systems (ES), integrated knowledge-belief base systems (IKBBS), automatic data capture (ADC), digital paper (DP), robotics, optical discs, etc.

These tools enable us to make an historic advance on Bacon's great Instauration - his reconstruction of knowledge.

Part of the problem can be understood by observing that each human brain needs to be educated ab initio to bring it up to date with its contemporary society's knowledge-belief, whereas each technologic advance is usually a marginal development of precursors.

As has been discussed above, the growth of global knowledge-belief has been so great that no individual human brain can record it all, let alone pass it on. Society's response to this problem is inadequate. Present approaches to achieving the necessary education are rudimentary. Many countries do not even have free basic or higher education.

In order to enable all humanity to reap the benefits of the Creation Revolution, there are many hurdles which mankind has had to leap in the quest to perceive and record knowledge-belief.

Some of the first knowledge-belief hurdles were the creation and use of tools, imitation, communication of a common sense, an understanding of action and transaction, demonstration, language, writing, quantification, mathematics, machines to improve upon our brains ability to perceive, e.g. scales (just noticeable differences [JND's]), telescopes, microscopes etc. More recent hurdles are printing via movable type (Gutenburg), photography, films, sound recording, etc. As the knowledge-belief revolution gained momentum, publication of knowledge-belief in loose leaf or microfiche enabled quicker updating. The recording of knowledge-belief in computer readable form (electronic publishing of information), the creation of the means to transfer human expertise to computers (expert systems), scanning tunnelling microscopes, the ability of humans to interact with and improve expert systems (interactive belief networks), the ability to link expert systems with machines (robotics), communal brains and world governmental regulation, are only some of the hurdles which have had to be leapt in the past or which remain for the future, in the quest to record knowledge-belief.

Each hurdle builds upon and includes the difficulties of previous ones.

The Knowledge-Belief Revolution in Health and Medicine

Medical knowledge-belief, in common with knowledge-belief as a whole, is in the midst of revolution. The explosion of knowledge-belief in general and medical knowledge-belief in particular, have meant that no individual can remember all. At present, all over the world, medical students attempt to learn medical knowledge-belief, how to access it and how to use it. During and after their medical studies they learn parts of the totality of medicine, but also they simultaneously forget parts.

In day to day medical practice, even if the practitioner does remember certain "facts", not all those "facts" will always be called to mind every time they are needed.

Computers and Computer Memory

Computers and computer memory have an important role to play in modern medicine. Recent developments in computer hardware, software, and information techniques such as the Unified Medical Language System (UMLS) coding systems e.g. Read code, SNOMED, SNOP, ICD-9 etc., knowledge-belief engineering, and distributed database have enabled us to begin to store and to use medical knowledge-belief in ways which are impossible for humans without the assistance of computers. Extreme care needs to be used in choosing and using systems of a classification, nomenclation, codification etc.

The demands on health professionals to obtain and apply more medical knowledge-belief are growing continuously. In parallel with this, the demands on health professionals to gather and report medical and non-medical information to various parts of the health system are also growing. Finally, health professionals are being asked to increase their efficiency in caring for patients.

To face these various and competing pressures, tools must be found to empower health professionals to satisfy the new and continuing demands being placed upon them while ensuring that the quality of medical care delivered to the patient not only does not deteriorate but improves.

Computer Tools for Manipulating Knowledge-Belief

In recent years computer technology and techniques have improved in ways which are directly relevant to problems facing health professionals. Among the most relevant improvements and developments are the following :

(i) the introduction of compact, flexible and powerful personal computers capable of operating at very high speed and priced low enough to be purchased for home and office use

(ii) the design of operating environments that provide simultaneous computer access to a large community of users and that allow users to share their knowledge-belief

(iii) interfaces between the user and the computer which use clear and intuitively understood metaphors which make the computer a transparent link between the user and the information

(iv) hardware, software, and knowledge-belief integration which enables information to be linked together in a variety of forms (e.g. text, data, sound, motion, knowledge-belief base) in order to maximise information access and transfer to the user.

(v) software engineering which enables computers to deliver the knowledge-belief, information manipulation and decision making skills of domain experts through less specialist intermediaries, e.g. knowledge-belief based systems

(vi) networks which can provide immediate and shared access to time - critical information

(vii) Portable, large capacity, robust and inexpensive information storage media :

An optical laser disc which is produced in a factory and can be read only and not written upon. This is called compact disc read only memory (CD-ROM) If several discs are used frequently they can be accessed more easily using a jukebox. Other optical technologies such as Compact Disk Interactive (CDI) and Digital Video Interactive (DVI) can provide full action video.

An optical laser disc which can be written on once and read many times is available. This is a called write once read many times disc (WORM) This produces an indelible record which is ideal for permanent patient records and other archives.

An optical laser disc which can be written on but this type of disc can be erased and written on many times as well as read many times. This is called a write many times read many times disc (WMRM).

The publication of the Oxford Textbook of Medicine OTM on CD-ROM is an early step in the progress of the electronic publishing of medical information. It is unfortunate that what could have been a value added product (VAP) is actually a value detracted product (VDP) since tables, figures and pictures which are in the paper version are not in the

CD-ROM version. Furthermore, no advantage has been taken of the multimedia potential of the CD-ROM. There are no graphics, motion graphics, photography, or sound etc. which now are possible with CD-ROMS.

The publication of the Oxford English Dictionary as a CD-ROM renders its complete contents available quickly to search for definitions, etymologies, etc. It is unfortunate that again no advantage was taken of the multimedia potential of CD-ROM; for example, archaic, phonetic symbols are retained while vocal pronunciation of the words is not included on a medium which was invented for sound i.e. CD-AUDIO.

Computer programmes enable us to link related "facts" which are on the patient record data card or disc. These links can be between related "facts" within a particular patient's record e.g. link a dental fact with a medical fact like allergy, and between hospital, dental, general practitioner, etc., record. Using "expert systems" we can link knowledge-belief about the specific individual patient and the general medical knowledge-belief base.

Qualitative and Quantitative Medicine

In order to make maximum use of the innovations of the knowledge-belief revolution we need both qualitative and quantitative information.

Qualitative Medicine
The clinician uses a wide and specialised vocabulary to express medical belief and knowledge-belief. Qualitative information is the norm in this vocabulary; quantitative expressions are less common.

At present medicine is taught, learned, and practiced primarily using qualitative descriptions of health and illness. For example, in discussing Kaposi's Sarcoma in AIDS, Pinching says "Kaposi's Sarcoma behaves as an opportunistic tumour that generally emerges in the host with defective cellular immunity, it is probably caused by a potentially oncogenic virus".

In just one sentence, four qualitative expressions are used viz, generally, defective, probably, and potentially. Each of these words refers to events which are countable and quantifiable.

The facilities available to medicine in the past have not been conducive to the collection of the quantitative information which is required to make the transition from medicine based on experience and subjective, qualitative information to medicine based on numbers (i.e. quantitative information).

It is questionable whether humans need or are even able, easily to use quantitative information in most health care provision. Obviously in the case of some procedures such as laboratory tests for electrolytes, blood gases, etc. we do use numbers. But most teaching, learning, and medical practice is more in line with the quotation from Pinching above. We use words like frequently, rarely, often, etc. The meanings of these words change, depending on the context of their semantic and syntactic fields. They reflect relative probabilities of knowing i.e. beliefs.

Humans are good at using qualitative terms, computers are not. Computers are best at manipulating quantified terms. In fact some computer programmes involving health care, use quantitative information and convert it into qualitative information for the human user.

The relative lack of importance of quantitative information for humans, and its importance for computers is forcibly made in the recent British Medical Journal series "Logic in Medicine".

Quantitative Medicine

Recent developments in Data Structure and Capture, Document Structure and Data Communications make it feasible for health professionals to capture patient records on the computer and to structure them. There are increasing needs for the development of standards for the representation of this data, the medical record, and the patient record. As these standards develop and complicated issues relating to the patient record as a database are studied and understood, the patient database may progressively provide a partial solution to the problem raised by Fox, vide supra.

As mentioned above, the patient record can be stored on Write Once Read Many times optical disks (WORM) while the patient is alive and the record needs updating. After death the same record can be stored on CD-ROM or its future replacement as an archival medium. This patient database is likely, progressively, to become what Fox refers to as a "source of reliable, quantitative parameters (symptom frequencies, resource costs, outcome costs) from which relative likelihoods or desirability of the decision option can be calculated". If we be correct in our prediction that the database will improve, then it will provide the source of quantitative health data which can be compared with already existing health knowledge-belief base. Such comparison will reinforce the knowledge-belief base if it be consistent with what is already known-believed or create new knowledge-belief if appropriate.

We refer to this approach to numerical analysis of linkages between symptoms, signs, diagnosis, treatment, prognosis, prevention etc., as Quantitative Medicine (QNM) to distinguish it from the past and present practice of Qualitative Medicine (QLM) which is not primarily numerical.

The practice of quantitative medicine will result in a far better understanding of diagnostic and therapeutic relationships and will be based on the actual practice of the medical practitioners themselves since their experiences will generate the statistics upon which quantitative medicine is based.

Recent literature related to computers and quantitative medicine date from 1959 when Ledley and Lusted published their seminal paper "Reasoning foundation of Medical

Diagnosis". They demonstrated how Baye's Theorem could be applied in a "live" medical setting. Their work on quantitative medicine has subsequently been followed by papers from others such as Card, Blum, Speigelhalter, Pearl, and Tversky, A.

Expert Systems and Knowledge-Belief Systems

Approaches to computing have been designed to help to overcome this qualitative - quantitative problem e.g. expert systems, knowledge-belief based systems etc.

Creating Knowledge-Belief Base From Experts

Judging from the expert systems, knowledge-belief bases and belief bases which have already been created in medical and other domains it is clear that it is feasible to create belief and knowledge-belief bases by collaboration of experts and knowledge-belief engineers.

Expert systems use both quantitative and qualitative information which is derived from experts, in order to design programmes which attempt to attain the same or a better quality of decision making compared with experts. In some cases the computer performance equals or surpasses that of the expert.

In creating expert systems, usually there are three main elements:

1. the expert who wishes to record his knowledge-belief as "facts" and "rules", i.e. elements of knowledge-belief;

2. a knowledge-belief engineer who is skilled at teasing out of the experts the "facts", "rules", etc. which enable them to exercise their judgments;

3. the computer hardware and software which are especially suited to represent knowledge-belief in expert systems.

Instead of using information by reading prose on paper, the computerised knowledge-belief base can be used by presenting an expert system with attributes of a problem or an opportunity. The expert system will then assemble the "facts" and "rules", etc., to suggest solutions similar to those which the expert(s) who created the belief and knowledge-belief base would have suggested.

The corpus of belief elements which represent the knowledge-belief in the system is referred to as a knowledge-belief base system (KBS). The transmission of a single element from one KBS to another we call a Belief Element Transmission (BET) unit. The quantification of the amount of belief transmitted must be judged relative to the transmitter and transmittee.

Creating Knowledge-Belief Base From Data Base
It is clear that a knowledge-belief base can be created from a data base. Take, for example, the case of thalidomide.

If the data base discussed above had been available when thalidomide was introduced, it would have been possible to observe quickly and easily that the observed number of neonatal malformations exceeded the expected number. The data base could then have been searched to find statistical associations to explain the increase in malformations.

The creation of knowledge-belief base from data base holds promise for the elicitation of the statistics necessary for developing quantitative medicine.

An approach to solving the problem of lack of quantitative information on which to base decisions has been made possible by the large scale introduction of computers into medical practice (vide supra).

The data bases which are being built up by medical information systems in operational use can be used for epidemiologic analysis, post marketing drug research and other market research, clinical trials, assessment of side effects, cost benefit analysis, morbidity surveys, resource management, etc. The availability of these computers, combined with a structured coding system and a computerised medical record may enable one to count the frequency of linkages between symptoms and signs and diagnoses. Work along these lines is described by Blum. These data bases will provide a massive amount of data on which one can attempt to establish quantitative medicine.

There are many potential problems which have to be overcome in the creation, use and analysis of these data bases. One of the most important is the need for a method of dealing with individual variations and differences between health professionals. This can be partially overcome by having a central core of general practices which can act as reference or "sentinel" practices, e.g. the Royal College of General Practitioners scheme in the UK, where the highest quality linkages can be ensured by double checking in collaboration with university research departments using double blind randomised control trials.

There are problems of bias inherent in any computerised system and its coding system. These must be considered in any analysis of the data base.

Another complementary approach is the use of statistical tests of significance to evaluate whether differences between and among practitioners and patients are important enough to effect the validity of the results of quantifying medicine.

Creating Knowledge-Belief Base From Information Base
Conventional information which is held on computer can also be analysed to extract the "facts" and "rules" which it contains (e.g. the ICL, Department of Health and Social Services Demonstrator). These "facts" and "rules" can be analysed and the knowledge-belief within them can then be represented as part of the knowledge-belief base.

Creating Larger Knowledge-Belief Base by the Integration of Separate Knowledge-Belief Bases

Data bases, information bases, and knowledge-belief bases can be broadened in their coverage by integrating two or more limited knowledge-belief bases. Standards need to be developed to enable those who are working on separate data bases, information bases, and knowledge-belief bases to have a common framework and standards to allow integration. National Health Services are often based on primary care and most patients are registered with a general practitioner. The general practitioner can refer patients to hospital consultants. The record of these encounters among patient, general practitioner, hospital consultant, and other health professionals results in the production of a data base on the health of the nation's population. At present most of this data is inaccessible because it is held on health professionals' paper records.

The increasing computerisation of these records is creating a data base on the health of nations (vide supra). The importance of this is that a computer held data base can be searched easily. New knowledge-belief can be created from the data base. These data bases are national assets of international significance.

International and National Organisations should be established to oversee and control the use of these Health Data Bases.

It was recognised, early in the creation of these national databases, when the amount of health information was held as very limited, that new knowledge-belief could be gained by linking episodes within patient's records. For example, the Oxford Record Linkage Study was established to exploit this potential.

Methodology for an Editorial Board Organisation for a Knowledge-Belief Base

Editorial boards are required to establish and to oversee common definitions (lexicons), common standards, knowledge-belief representation techniques, a common framework, consistency checkers, belief maintenance, and "provable correctness". The editorial board should also update and maintain the knowledge-belief base. Research into the integration and maintenance of knowledge-belief based systems must be seen as a legitimate and urgent issue.

The Editorial Board-in-Chief comprise members of each of the main domains of interest e.g. health, publishing, information, national and international governmental bodies, the commercial sector etc. The sectors of the Editorial Board-in-Chief also meet separately.

The content of the World Health Knowledge-belief Base is divided into major categories and is subdivided to create knowledge-belief base domains which are manageable by Editorial Boards; standards setting, validation; major categories of activity such as the belief domain itself, management of the belief domain, education and research, and specific diseases such as AIDS, Rabies etc.

Integration of Knowledge-Belief Systems

The development of knowledge-belief based systems standards will enable collaborating groups to integrate their knowledge-belief bases. A group has been set up to attempt to do this on an international scale. It has proposed a set of rules, the Arden Syntax, that may allow belief elements to be mapped from one system to another. A study of the legal consequences of the use of single knowledge-belief based systems and integrated ones is a high priority of the European Community Advanced Informatics in Medicine (AIM) programme and also of the USA Food and Drug Administration.

Global Issues

In this section we wish to highlight some major issues which were raised in the Working Group as items of major concern for IMIA, global bodies, regional bodies, national bodies, and especially, learned colleges and boards of all the various health professions. The World Health Organisation itself uses information technology and management information in order to improve management techniques at global headquarters, regional and national level; it commissioned a report of this aspect of its own use of information technology.

Independent, in depth, professional analysis and reports are required at all levels to enable the information technologists and commercial interests to work together with health professionals in the interests of patients. We must develop professionally responsible, ethically and morally acceptable practices. The same or higher standards must be set in the use of information technology in pursuit of health as are set for the "ethical" drug industry.

Eternal vigilance is the price of professional freedom from domination by bureaucrats, information technicians, and commercial bad practice.

Information Systems and Services Acquisition Methodology

Careful attention must be paid to the application of rigorous and methodical acquisition of information systems and services.
Various information systems acquisition methodologies have been proposed. None is ideal and few standards exist.

One cause of this problem is that humans take information for granted in their non - professional lives. This leads often to a nonchalance about information standards in their professional lives.

In building a hospital, the client is expected to draw up a brief stating requirements; an architect is required to draw up plans to achieve them; and to supervise building, a quantity surveyor should do a detailed survey of quantities; and many other professional activities are required to produce the building which would allow the client to carry out the functions and tasks which should be identified in the original brief of requirements. One would not build a hospital without such a brief and blueprints. Just such rigour is required in the building of information systems and services, especially where defects will threaten patients' lives. Yet for the reasons stated above, the requirement for employment of a system acquisition methodology is more honoured in the breach than in the observance. As Blois observed - we lack adequate theoretical foundations, conceptual structures, and principles to guide the introduction of information technology into health care.

As a beginning "ABC" toward a system acquisition methodology (SAM), we suggest the following:

Accept the need for, commission, and fund the introduction of information technology into health care at all levels. Accept the results of the plan as a programme per se in a programme budgeting system. Establish criteria for evaluation and assessment of quality and quantity for each phase of the programme. Insist on the best available standards for formal Logical Representation Techniques (LRT), mathematical provability, and "truth" and belief maintenance.

Budget for all stages of the development of the system right from the start of strategic planning and program budgeting to the continuing maintenance and updating of the information system and service. This may sound obvious but in our experience, it is hardly ever done properly.

Control the development of the information system and service. Regular meetings of a quality assurance (QA) group should be held. The group should use one of the recognised formal methodologies.

Develop the system plan using a "top down" approach in which a group of user representatives works with the system developers to create an overall strategy which will ensure that the system can be comprehensive and integrated. Implement the system plan using a "bottom up" approach in which the information providers are involved, if possible, on an individual or small group basis. The system should be designed so that, as far as possible, the information is captured during the patient encounter and provides immediate utility and feedback to the patient and the health professional.

Evaluate the development, implementation, maintenance, and updating of the information system and service. The user representative group or a quality assurance group comprising users who are not members of the user representative group should agree a regular programme to evaluate the degree to which the strategic plan and implementation plans are being met. It should be accepted that the maintenance and updating process is continuous. This involves periodic re-evaluation of the changes in the tasks and functions of the users of the system and changes and developments in the information "environment" which may enhance the service.

Global Free Software
The commercial nature of computer software is an interesting one. The initial effort to transform an idea for a computer function into software is usually expensive, difficult, and time consuming. Once there is an initial implementation of the idea, it is usually less expensive, less difficult and less time consuming to imitate it, and often programmers eventually produce software which is "free" or nearly free for one reason or another (e.g. the shareware system in the United States and Europe and the free software which is made available through the World Health Organisation).

The availability of this "freeware" creates opportunities and problems - especially in the poorer countries of the world. The greatest opportunity is that for technology transfer, which is one of WHO's major missions. WHO can make available a few types of free software e.g. EPIINFO which was developed by the Centres for Disease Control (CDC) in the United States. This has been adopted and adapted in many countries.

EPIINFO is designed to allow easy construction of forms and questionnaires for disease surveillance. These forms and questionnaires, when filled in, create a data base. EPIINFO has other modules which analyse the database, do statistical calculations, draw graphs, and import and export data bases. EPIINFO is available free.

Immediate Implications for Public Health

(i) Opportunities
There are immediate implications of the wide scale computerisation of personal health records. Many hospital and general practice systems have built in telephones (modems) or other links to communication networks. Using these communication links, elements of the personal record can be communicated among health professionals. (Technical solutions to data protection and confidentiality must be employed). These types of links are referred to as electronic shared care.

A number of computerisation projects are being pursued in order to use electronic shared care to improve individual and public health (eg Minitel in France). At the Warwick University Expert System and Decision Support Unit, we are developing one which has immediate and practical implications for public health in relation to notifiable diseases. Globally, registered medical practitioners are required by law to notify certain diseases (see Global Sanitary Conventions of the United Nations and the World Health Organisation). In most countries, it is a criminal offence not to notify these diseases.

Nevertheless, notification rates are very low. For example, the notification rate for tetanus in the UK is 33%. This is explained more fully in (OPCS (1986)).

We have tagged all notifiable diseases in the Read code. The strike of the key which attributes a notifiable disease to a patient, automatically triggers a mechanism which sends the information which is required by statute, to the computer of the legal "proper officer".

In most cases this is either the Medical Officer of Environmental Health (MOEH), the Consultant in Communicable Disease Control (CCDC), or the Chief Environmental Health Officer (CEHO). The automation of notification of these diseases creates the possibility of collecting, automatically, non - aggregated and aggregated data on morbidity, mortality, and lifestyle. This aggregate data base is a national and international asset. It can be used for epidemiological purposes and for creating new medical knowledge-belief.

We have linked automatic notification of notifiable diseases to EPIINFO and other data bases. Thus the disease surveillance process can be speeded up from a matter of weeks to one of hours.

This data base and those related to other health states can also be used for management of health services at local, national and international level. At all these levels, there are increasing reports of a growing consensus that in order to improve health and to control costs, health service management and its management information systems need to be improved.

By negotiation it is possible to extend the data shared between medical practitioners and consultants in public health to all morbidity data via, for example, EPINET, the epidemiologic computer communications network.

(ii) Problems
EPIINFO also illustrates some of the problems with free software. As stated above, information systems, software, and hardware need planning and continual updating. There also should be support for users in the form of continuing training and education, and a telephone help-line. In many countries in which EPIINFO is being used, this support is inadequate or non existent. Protection against the introduction of computer viruses is negligently absent in most systems. There are other free systems such as the Peru Pharmaceutical database. We feel that these issues concerning public domain software, "shareware", and other "free" systems should be established on a more formal basis at a global, regional and national level, in fulfillment of the WHO remit to facilitate global technology transfer.

As described above, many information systems are developed without adequate control of the development, its quality, and standards by the ultimate users of the system. This has been a major cause of failure in system implementation.

Management and Management Information Systems
Management and management information are increasingly being seen as a continuing process involving four major steps (PACE) :
- P Identification and measurement of Problems and Opportunities;

- A Identification of Alternative Solutions;

- **C** Selection of the optimum alternative solution on the basis of Cost Benefit Analysis.

- **E** Evaluation of the implementation of the chosen solution in terms of its achievement of objectives.

This problem - opportunity cycle can be applied, in principle, to most management tasks. It also provides a basis for function analysis and information requirements upon which a system specification can be based. Simulation models make it possible to make projections on which dynamic management decisions can be made on subjects as diverse as resources for an accident and emergency department, the management of a threat of a rabies outbreak, to the health effects of the global population explosion, and global pollution such as warming etc.

International Standards For Health Information Services
Some national strategic plans (e.g. 5 year master plans) for health informatics make provision for national standard setting bodies for health information systems and services.

The universe of information technology started with no standards. Pioneers such as Von Neumann, Shannon, Turing, Hodges, etc, explored the underlying principles of information technology and suggested standards which seemed to be the most effective and efficient at the time e.g. setting threshold voltages to indicate logical truth and falsehood, and methods for combining sets of such logical states.

Since that time many standards for information technology have been established. The British Standards Institute (BSI) was the first national standards body in the world. There are now more than 80 similar organisations which belong to the International Standards Organisation (ISO) and International Electrotechnical Commission (IEC).

Unfortunately in the world of health information, few standards exist for recording and transmitting data, information, and knowledge-belief.

It is important that the issue of standards be addressed by the global, regional and national colleges and learned bodies of the health professions themselves. Appropriate organisational structures to create and maintain such standards should be established and supported financially.

An area which should be singled out for urgent attention is that of standard setting for decision support, expert systems and knowledge - belief systems. Some present day decision support systems, especially those on the subject of drug interactions are defective. There are many historic precedents related to standards for drugs and drug information (Ref Data Sheet Compendium). National and International Committees on the safety and quality control of decision support are required urgently to establish and maintain professional standards.

Quality Control and Audit
A corollary of standard setting is the creation of organisational structures which audit and control the quality of systems which aspire to achieve the standards. This is a matter for the health professions.

Escrow
Many health information systems are being developed by the commercial organisations whose primary motive is profit. It is of global and national importance that centres should be established with which the source codes of all systems containing patient records are lodged. Data Protection Acts should establish that all developers of these clinical systems should be required by law to deposit their source code (in escrow) with an approved centre. This would ensure that if a company were to go bankrupt or if a system failed, the approved centre would know sufficient to enable it to save and transfer the patient records and protect the data. We know of at least one course which gives guidance on this issue (Legal Studies and Services Ltd (1990)).

Cost Benefit Analysis
Three studies (de Dombal, F. (1974), de Dombal, F. (1986), Pritchard, P. (1986)) have concluded that the savings which would result from widespread use of expert systems in health would warrant Departments of Health giving a health expert system to all doctors.

In these studies, only the savings in prescribing costs and other "process costs" were analysed and on that basis alone the expert systems under study would result in massive savings. These studies did not attempt to analyse the cost savings from improved decision making in other cost areas, nor were the benefits in improved health evaluated.

It is clear that if the systems are justified on drug and process cost savings alone then they should be shown to be far more cost beneficial when all costs and benefits are included. Research to create adequate expert systems should be encouraged and supported financially in order to take advantage of the potential of expert systems in achieving these health benefits and in controlling the escalating costs of health care.

Conclusion

The consequences of the new information technology for the practice of medicine is only beginning to dawn on society. At the date of publishing this paper, it is disappointing to note that one of the latest publications on the relationship amongst culture, health, and illness appears to make no reference to the implications of the introduction of information technology to health. It will not be long before patients will have portable health data cards or discs holding general practitioner records, hospital records, etc. which can interact with a multimedia medical knowledge-belief base (including films, video, moving and still graphics, pictures and diagrams). These record systems will enable communication among Family Practitioner Committees, Health Authorities, Public Health Laboratory Services,

Communicable Diseases Surveillance Centres, and equivalent organisations etc. both nationally and internationally.

There are many advantages for both patients and health professionals, which are inherent in the knowledge-belief
revolution. Health problems will be dealt with more effectively. A large part of the total health knowledge-belief base will be available to health professionals. And last but not least, the use of the tools of the knowledge-belief revolution will result in health care at a lower cost.

Our role as physicians is to help individuals maintain and improve their health. Community physicians have a special responsibility for the health of communities.

As has been made abundantly clear throughout the history of civilisation all elements of the universe relate to each other. This universal relativity and wholeness may be violated in processes in some sectors of energy-space-time-order in physical and/or biological realms, but such dislocations are inherently unstable. A stable process will eventually emerge, but it is unlikely to bear much resemblance to its previous self because the evolution of the universe will have progressed.

This paper has discussed the creation revolution which is taking place on earth. It remains to be seen whether the tools of the creation revolution can be developed and harnessed to save our ecology from the simultaneous destruction revolution which is also taking place on earth. There are limits to growth and there are laws of universal relativity which can not be violated with impunity.

References

Abrett, G. Burstein, M. (1988). The KREME knowledge editing environment. In : Knowledge - Based Systems, Vol. 2. Academic Press Ltd.

Aligheri, D. (1310). De Monarchia.

Apperson, G., Doherty, R. Displaying Images. In : Zoellick, B. (Ed). CD-ROM - optical publishing. Microsoft Books.

Apple Computer Corporation (1987). HyperCard User's Manual (1987). Cupertino, Ca.

Avnir, D. (1989). The Fractal Approach to Heterogenous Chemistry. Surfaces, Colloids, Polymers. Wiley.

Baccaria, C. (1804). Elementi di Economica Pubblica.

Bacon, F. (begun 1610b). Instauratio Magna. Bacon, F. (1610a). Novum Organum.

Bacon, F. (begun 1610b). Instauratio Magna. Bacon, F. (1610c). Wisdom of the Ancients.

Baldwin, J., Acheson, E., Graham, W. (1987). Textbook of Medical Record Linkage. Oxford Medical Publications.

Barnett, O., Winickogg, R. (1990). Quality Assurance and Computer Based Patient Records. American Journal of Public Health Medicine, May 1990, Vol.80, No.5

Bayes, T. (1763). An essay towards solving a problem in the doctrine of chances. Phil. Trans. 3:370-418. Reproduced in Two Papers by Bayes, ed. W.E. Deming. New York : Hafner (1963).

Bell, D. (1974). - The Coming of Post Industrial Society - A Venture in Social Forecasting.

Belsnes, D., Moller-Pedersen, B. (1989). On a reference model for health care information processing and communication, and its implementation in ODA. Norwegian Computing Centre, Oslo, Norway.

Berg, B., Paris - Roth, J. (1989). Software for Optical Storage. Meckler Publishing.

Bergson, H. (1907). L' evolution creatrice. Bibliotheque de philosophie contemporanne, Paris.

Berkeley, G. (1709). An Essay towards a New Theory of Vision. Berkeley, G. (1721). De Motu.

Berkeley, G. (1730). Three Dialogues between Hylas and Philonous. Blois, M. (1984). Information and Medicine. The Nature of Medical Descriptions. University of California Press.

Blum, R. (1982). Discovery and Representation of Causal Relationships from a large time - oriented database : The RX Project. Sprnger Verlag.

Bradshaw, K. et al. (1984). Physician Decision Making - Evaluation of data used in a computerised ICU. International Journal of Clinical Monitoring and Computing, 1, 81 - 91.

Brewer, T. (1985). Developing and Implementing a systems strategy. Butler Cox.

British Standards Institute. Catalog 1990. Milton Keynes.

Brittain, R., Hurrion, R., McMorran, S., McMorran, J., Gupta, R. (1988a). An Expert Advisory System for the Acquired Immunodeficiency Syndrome (AIDS). Medical Informatics : Computers in Clinical Medicine. London : British Medical Informatics Society, 133 - 9.

Brittain, R. (1981). State of Bahrain, Ministry of Health, National Health Information Systems and Services Strategic Plan.

Brittain, R. (1988). An Editorial Board for the development of Knowledge Based Systems. North Warwickshire District Health Authority.

Brittain, R. Universal Relativity (Completed 1968). A Concept Unifying Physical and Biologic Relativity. Presented to the AAAS (1971) and published in Reviews on Environmental Health, Vol.III, No.2, 1980.

Brittain, R. (1989). Consultant aupres de l 'OMS, Royaume du Maroc, Ministere de la Sante Publique, Plan Directeur Quinquennal D '

Informatique Pour Le Systeme National de l'Information et de la Gestion Sanitaires.

Brittain, R., Hurrion, R., McMorran, J., Gupta, R., McMorran, S. (1988b). An Expert Advisory System for AIDS. In : Duru, G., Englebrecht, R., Flagle, C., Van Elmeren, W. (Eds.). La Science des Systems dans le domaine de la sante. No. 140. Collection de Medecine Legale et de Toxicologie Medicale.

Brittain, R. (1981). World Health Organisation, Geneva, Report on the World Health Organisation Information System.

Brittain, R. (1971). International Inequality. Task Force 1. In : Proceedings of the National House Staff Conference. St. Louis, Missouri. United States Department of Health Education and Welfare.

Brittain, R., McMorran, S. Principia Fidei et Communis Sensus. (Paper version in Press).

Brittain, R., McMorran, S. (1990). Principia Fidei et Communis Sensus. CD-PEDIA Series. Nimbus Records.

Brown, J., Vallbona, C. (1988). A New Patient Record Using the Laser Card. In : Proceedings of the Twelfth Symposium on Computer Applications in Medical Care, Washington. IEEE Press.

Burrows, J. (1968). Darwin : The Origin of Species. Penguin.

Bush, V. (1945). "As we may think". Atlantic Monthly, 101 - 108.

Campbell, D., Marciniak, T., Srivastava, S. (1988). The WORM in Research. In : Proceedings of the Twelfth Symposium on Computer Applications in Medical Care, Washington. IEEE Press.

Card, W. (1967). Towards A Calculus of Medicine. Medical Annual, 8 - 21.

Centres for Disease Control (1990). EPIINFO - Users Manual. USD Inc.

Clark, G., Sohn, D. (1966), World Peace Through World Government. Harvard Press. Third Edition.

Clayton, P., Pryor, T., Wigertz, O., Hripcsak, G. (1989). Issues and Structures for Sharing Medical Knowledge Among Decision Making Systems : The 1989 Arden Homestead Retreat. In : Proceedings of the Thirteenth Symposium on Computer Applications in Medical Care (SCAMC), Washington. IEEE Computer Society Press.

Clayton, P., Pryor, A., Wigertz, O., Johnson, S., Hripcsak, G. (1988). Sharing Medical Knowledge for Automated Decision-making. In : Proceedings of the Twelfth Symposium on Computer Applications in Medical Care, Washington. IEEE Press.

CMC Research Inc. (1989). Shakespeare on Disc.

Conklin, J. (1987). "Hypertext : An Introduction and Survey". IEEE Computer, 20, (9), 17 - 41.

College of American Pathologists (1965). SNOP : Systematised Nomenclature of Pathology. Skokie, Ill.

Cornelia, V. (1986). Information Technology : Value for Money.

Cote, R. (1982). Systematized Nomenclature of Medicine. Skokie, Ill.: College of American Pathologists.

Crombie, D., Fleming, D., Norbury, C. (1989). Weekly Returns Service. Report for 1988. Royal College of General Practitioners Research Unit, Birmingham.

de Dombal, F. et al. (1986). Computer Aided Diagnosis of acute abdominal pain : a multicentre study. British Medical Journal, 293.

de Dombal, F., Horrocks, J. (1974). Computer Aided Diagnosis: conclusions from an overall experience involving 4449 patients. In : Anderson, J., and Forsythe, J. (Eds). MEDINFO 1974, North Holland.

Department of Health and Human Services (1980). International Classification of Diseases (9th revision, clinical modification). Bethseda, Md. (DHSS publication no. (PHS) 80-1260).

Department of Health (1990). N.H.S. Review. Working for Patients. Framework for Information Systems. I.T. Consultative Document Comprising Recommendations of the Department Review Program 25 on Informatics.

Dowey, J., Elstein, A. (1988). Professional Judgement. Cambridge.

Down, S., Walker, M., Blum, R. (1986). Automated summary of on -line medical records. In : Proceedings of MEDINFO - 86, Washington.

Dubois, P. (1306). De Recupertione Terrae Sanctae.

Dubos, R. (1965). Man adapting. Yale U.P.

Dunwoodie, D. (1985). Diagnostic Systems. In : Sheldon, M., Stoddart, M. (Eds). Trends in General Practice Computing. Royal College of General Practitioners.

Einberger, J., Zoellick, B. (1986). CD-ROM. Vol. 2, Optical Publishing. Microsoft Press.

Einstein, A. (1915). Relativity. The Special and the General Theory. University Paperbacks.

Engelbart, D., English, W. (1968). A Research Centre for Augmenting Human Intellect. AFIPS Conf. Proc., Vol.33, Part 1, The Thompson Book Company, Washington.

Erasmus, D. (1514). Querela Pacis and other writings.

Erickson, P., Henke, K-D., Brittain, R. (1981). A Health Statistics Framework : US Data Systems as a model for European Health Information. In : Culyer, A. (Ed). (1981). A Report to the British Social Science Research Council and the European Science Foundation. Institute of Social and Economic Research, University of York.

European Econonomic Community (1988). Advanced Informatics in Medicine initiative. FDA.

Fielding, T. (1987). CD ROM, Blueprint Publishing Ltd.

Final Report of the GMSC/RCGP Joint Computing Technical Working Party, The Classification of General Practice, GMSC August 1988

Forrester, J. (1971). World Dynamics. Wright Allen Press.

Fox, J. (1985a). Artificial Intelligence in Medicine (Artificial Intelligence in Primary Care). North - Holland.

Fox, J. (1985b). Judgement, Policy and the Harmony Machine, Imperial Cancer Research Fund Laboratories. Proceedings of the International Joint Conference on Artificial Intelligence 1985

Fox, J., Glowinski, A., O'Neill, M. (1987). The Oxford System of Medicine : A prototype for Primary Care. In : AIME 87 : Proceedings of the International Conference on Artificial Intelligence in Medicine, Marseilles. Lecture Notes in Medical Informatics, Springer Verlag.

Fulton, J. (1988). X - Window System, Ver. 11, Rel. 3. MIT.

Garrison, F. (1929). History of Medicine. W.B. Saunders.

Giuse, N., Giuse, D., Miller, R. (1989). Medical Knowledge Base Construction as a means of Introducing Students to Medical Informatics. In : Proceedings of the International Symposium of Medical Informatics in Education, Victoria, B.C., Canada.

Glass, L., Mackey, M. (1988). Clocks to Chaos. Rhythms of Life. Princeton University Press.

Goldberg, D. (1990). Genetic Algorithms : In Search, Optimisation and Machine Learning. Addison Wesley.

Gordon, B. (1971). Ed. : Current Medical Information and Terminology, 4th edition, American Medical Association, Chicago, 1971.

Grolier Electronic Publishing, Inc. (1989). The New Grolier Electronic Encylopedia (1989).

Gunton, T. (1983). Strategic Systems Planning, Report 34, March 1983. Butler Cox.

Handy, C., The Future of Work - Guide to a Changing Society 1984. Basil Blackwell Publishing Inc.

Hargrave, L., Hutchinson, A., Cavill, A., Goldstone, L., Watson, H. (1988). Computerised Family Practitioner Records - a database for General Practitioners. J. Roy. Coll. Gen. Pract., 1988. 38. 22-23.

Harman, P. (1982). Energy, Force and Matter. The Conceptual Development of Nineteenth - Century Physics. Cambridge University Press.

Helman, C. (1990). Culture, Health and Illness, 2nd Edition. Wright, London.

Hodges, A. (1983). Alan Turing. The Enigma of Intelligence. Unwin.

House of Commons (1987). Third Report to Social Services

Select Committee, Session 1986-7. Problems Associated with AIDS. HMSO, London.

Humphreys, B., Lindberg, D. (1989). Building the Unified Medical Language System (UMLS). In : Proceedings of the Thirteenth

Symposium on Computer Applications in Medical Care (SCAMC), Washington. IEEE Computer Society Press.

Information Management Centre of the National Health Service (1990). Logical Representation Techniques.

Jones, W.H.S. (1923). The Hippocratic Writings, 4 Vols, Loeb Classics, New York.

Kant, I. (1795). Zum ewigen Frieden.

Laub, L. (1988). Information Delivery Systems. In : Zoellick, B. (Ed). CD-ROM - optical publishing. Microsft Books.

Ledley, R., Lusted, L. (1959). Reasoning Foundations of Medical Diagnosis. Science, 130 : 9 - 21.

Legal Studies and Services Ltd. (1990). Negotiating Computer Contracts. Practical Computing, April 1990.

Logie, K. (1986). The Alphabet Affect. William Morrow Inc.

Lough, J. (1954). The Encyclopedie of Diderot and D'Alembert. Cambridge.

Lowe, H., Barnett, G. (1987). MicroMeSH : a microcomputer system for exploring the National Library of Medicine's Medical Subject Headings Vocabulary. In : Proceedings of the Eleventh Symposium on Computer Applications in Medical Care, Washington. IEEE Press.

Mach, E. (1890). Contributions to the Analysis of the Sensations. Open Court Classics.

Malthus, R. (1797). An Essay on Population.

Matheson and Cooper (1982). Academic Information Management in the Academic Health Sciences Centre.

McMorran, J. (1989). An Expert Advisory System for AIDS. Ph.D. Thesis. University of Warwick.

McMorran, S. (1986). An Expert System for Rabies. M.Sc. Thesis, University of Warwick.

McMorran, S. (1988). Expert Systems in Medicine - the reasons for their successes and failures, and suggestion as to how they should be taken further. Report to the Winston Churchill Trust, London.

Meadows, D., Meadows, D. (1970). Limits to Growth. MIT Press.

Meckler Corp. (1988). Optical Information Systems (1988). Buyers Guide and Consultant Directory.

Mesarovic, M., Pestel, E. (1975). Mankind at the Turning Point. The Second Report to the Club of Rome. Hutchinson.

Miller, P., Ball, S., Kidd, K. (1989). The Human Gene Mapping Library Database : Representational Challenges Posed by New Bioscience Technologies and by Evolving Biomedical Knowledge. In : Proceedings of the Thirteenth Symposium on Computer Applications in Medical Care, Washington. IEEE Press.

Miller, R., McNeil, M., Challinor, S. et al. (1986). The INTERNIST - 1 / QUICK MEDICAL REFERENCE Project - Status Report. Western Journal of Medicine, 145, 816 - 822.

Miller, R., Masarie, F., Myers, J. (1986). Quick Medical Reference (QMR) for diagnostic assistance. M.D. Computing 3(5):34-48.

Morgan, C. (1986). Inside XENIX. Howard W. Sams, Indianapolis.

Morris, P. (1987). Modelling Cognition. Wiley.

Murray, K. (1978). Caught in the Web of Words. Yale University Press.

Nakau, M., Axeland, S. (1983). Numbers are better than words. Verbal specification of frequency have no place in medicine. The American Journal of Medicine, 74, 1061 - 1065.

Nayemi-Rad, F., Koschmann, T., Lee, C., Kepic, T., Evens, M. (1988). Maintaining a Knowledge Base Using the MEDAS Knowledge Engineering Tools. In :Proceedings of the Ninth Symposium on Computer Applications in Medical Care, Washington. IEEE Press.

OPCS Monitor. MB 2 - 86 - 1. Government Statistical Service.

Organick, E. (1972). The Multics System : An Examination of its Structure. MIT Press, Cambridge, MA.

OUP (1987). The Oxford English Dictionary on Compact Disc (1987).

Owl International, Inc. (1987). Guide Reference Manual (1987). Bellevue, WA.

Paine, T. (1801). The Maritime Contract.

Parry, P. (1978). OXMIS codes. Oxford Regional Health Authority.

Pearl, J. (1986c). Fusion, propagation and structuring in belief networks. Artificial Intelligence 29, 3, 241 - 88.

Phillips, C. (1988). Logic in Medicine, British Medical Journal

Pinching, A.J. (1986). Clinics in Immunology and Allergy Volume 6/Number 3, October.

Pylyshn, Z. (1986). Computation and Cogniton. Toward a foundation for cognitive science. MIT Press.

Read, J. (1986). Computer Coding - British Journal of Health Care Computing May 1986.

Recommendation X3.131 (1986). The Small Computer Systems Interface. American National Standards Institute (ANSI).

Reichertz, P. (1987). Preparing for change : concepts and education in medical informatics. Computer Methods and Programs in Biomedicine, 25, 89 - 102.

Report of the Board of Regents, National Library of Medicine U.S. Department of Health and Human Services, Long Range Plan, January 1987.

Ritchie, D. (1984). The Evolution of the UNIX Time Sharing System. AT&T Bell Laboratories Technical Journal, Oct. 1984, Vol. 63, No. 8, Part 2, 1577-1594.

Robertson, J. (1905). Philosophical Works. London.

Runes, D. (1963). Pictorial History of Philosophy. Littlefield, Adams and Co., Pattison, New Jersey.

Rutkowska, J., Crook, C. (1987). Computers, Cognition and Development. Issues for Pyschology and Education. Wiley.

Sandness, J. (1989). Use of Online Databases by Practicing Physicians. In : Proceedings of the Thirteenth Symposium on Computer Applications in Medical Care, Washington. IEEE Press.

Sargent, M., Shoemaker, R. (1984). The IBM Personal Computer From the Inside Out. Addison - Wesley, Publishing Company.

Shannon, C., Weaver, W. (1949). The Mathematical Theory of Communication. University of Illinois Press.

Sheldon, N. , Stoddart, N. (1985). Trends in General Practice Computing. Royal College of General Practitioners.

Shortliffe, E. (1976). Computer Based Medical Consultation. MYCIN. Elsevier / North Holland.

Shryock, R. (1961). In : Quantification. A History of the Meaning and Measurement in the Natural and Social Sciences. Bobbs Merrill Company, Inc.

Smith, D. (1987). Performance Indicators in General Practice. In : Gray, D. (Ed). Medical Annual 1987, 202-208.

Smith, J., Stutely, R. (1988). SGML. The Users Guide to ISO 8879. Ellis Horwood.

Smith, F., Miller, G. (1966). The Genesis of Language - a psycholinguistic approach. MIT Press.

Smith, W., Hahn, J. (1989). Hypermedia or Hyperchaos :Using HyperCard To Teach Medical Decision Making. In : Proceedings of the Thirteenth Symposium for Computer Applications in Medicine, Washington. IEEE Computer Press.

Sorabji, R. (1988). Matter, Space and Motion. Theories in Antiquity and their Sequel. Duckworth.

Spiegelhalter D., Knill-Jones R. (1984). Statistical and Knowledge Based Approaches to Clinical Decision support Systems, with an Application in Gastroenterology. (Reprinted from The Journal of the Royal Statistical Society Series A volume 147 Part 1 1984)

Spivey J. (1988). Understanding Z - A Specification Language and its Formal Semantics, Cambridge University Press.

Stevens, R. (1988). Experiments with Computer Card Medication Records in Britain. In : Proceedings of International Conference and Workshop on Smart Card Applications and Technologies. Peterborough. PLF Commun 1988 : 12.

Taylor, D. (1984). Understanding the NHS in the 1980's. Office of Health Economics, London.

The Foreign Office (1990). Web of Care. A video commissioned by the Foreign Office and produced by the Central Office for Information, London.

Turing, A. (1956). Can Machines Think ? The World of Mathematics. Ed. Newman, J. Simon and Schuster, New York.

Tuttle, M. et. al. (1989). Implementing Meta - 1. The First Version of the UMLS Metathesaurus. In : Proceedings of Thirteenth Symposium for Computer Applications in Medical Care, Washington. IEEE Computer Society Press.

Tversky, A., Kahneman, D. (1980). Causal Schemas in Judgments about Uncertainty. In : Fishbein, M. (Ed). Progress in Social Psychology. Hillsdale. Jolla, Ca.

United Nations (1990). United Nations Population Fund Report, 19, the State of World Population.

United Nations Intergovernmental Panel on Climatic Change (1990). United Nations Plaza, New York.

University of Latter Day Saints Hospital (1988). HELP - a snapshot through time.

Urmson, J. (1982). Berkeley. Past Masters Series. Oxford University Press.

Von Neumann, J. (1958), The Computer and the Brain. Yale University Press.

Walker, M., Blum, R. (1986). Towards automated discovery from clinical databases : The RADIX Project. In : Proceedings of MEDINFO - 86, Washington.

Wallace, A. (1870). Theory of Natural Selection.

Weatherall D.J., Ledingham J.G.G., Warrell, D.A. (1989a). Oxford Textbook of Medicine Second Edition (CD-ROM Version). Oxford University Press.

Weatherall D.J., Ledingham J.G.G., Warrell, D.A. (1989b). Oxford Textbook of Medicine Second Edition (Paper Version). Oxford University Press.

Wellbank, M., Knowledge Acquisition for Expert Systems : A Review

of techniques, British Telecom Research Laboratories, Martlesham, Ipswich 1983.

Wells, H. G. (1933). The Shape of the things to come. McMillan Press.

Wells, H.G. (1932). The Work, Wealth and Happiness of Mankind. Heinemann.

Williams, T. (1989). Optical storage inches towards standards. Computer Design, Oct., 1989. Discs.

Winfree, A. (1987). When Time Breaks Down. Princeton University Press.

World Health Organisation (1988). Informatics and Telematics in Health. Present and Potential Uses. Geneva.

World Health Organisation. The World Health Organisation Oath Declaration of Geneva, [1948; Sydney, 1968;].

Wynner, E., Lloyd, G. (1946). Searchlight on Peace Plans. E.P. Dutting and Company.

International Primary Care Computing
G.M. Hayes and N. Robinson (Editors)
Elsevier Science Publishers B.V. (North-Holland)
© IMIA, 1991

7.2 SECOND DISCUSSANT

Dr Rupert Fawdry

We need to consider what is practical in "Third World" terms. There is no such thing as an "expert" in this field at present. We cannot influence the way in which it goes. We can communicate trends or notice trends but influencing it has very little effect. Imagining that there can be a Third World IT technique is not feasible.

We need to touch on the few areas where we can meet and have influence and to concentrate our efforts onto practical implementations such as word processors. There is a need to make use of the best possible technology and not to be too general or specific.

GENERAL DISCUSSION.

There is a fear of IT. This fear, a personal and cultural fear applies to GPs in this country. Eskimos can use computers as they are a very adaptable people. We need to help encourage the forward movement of individuals in this field. The human mind has the ability to use the machine. Uses of computers should be encouraged, rather than discouraged by whoever, even if it leads to some being unused. It does allow human beings to improve the quality of their life. Such a quantum leap should be made available to everyone.

TV distribution was prior to satellite and now some governments wish that radios were not able to distribute information to the bush. The quantum leap could go in a different direction and be used as a powerful source of information for the government. We should see the possibilities of giving health care professionals cheap tools, which are simple, with programs which support key things happening.

A good example are the Olivetti machines distributed via WHO mainly for monitoring growth and development of children and others. We need to identify possible dangers, e.g. Rumania and the Securitate if they had access to information.
Local influences may be limited eg even near the capital, Freetown of Sierra Leone, it is not possible to receive local radio, while the BBC World Service can be received. Similarly, TV, except in the few countries where it is possible for them to generate their own programmes, usually has to be bought in from elsewhere producing a new cultural imperialism.

With IT this will happen again and there will be a need to buy in. In India they are creating their own software, so things are happening, but there are reasons for ensuring that local expertise needs to be generated. Resources are becoming available eg. huge databases.

99% of Third World IT is out of control, but for the remaining 1% we should try to make sure that what is available is appropriate.

Control must be exerted over decision support in health computing. Recommend quality support of knowledge-based and decision support systems.

Need to improve access to care and information needed. Can we recommend sources where information is available?

Information sessions available here are only in the foetal stage eg computerising Chinese Medicine.

There is a large amount of information in the world and people need to be able to get access to it and see what health systems are available elsewhere.

OR In Harare, Zimbabwe there are simple recording techniques for health care management eg, just measuring cervical size, being used to train traditional health workers. Pictorial representation is used. This does need to be evaluated.

There is a need to evaluate ideas and test them in the real environment as these can be unsuitable, if technique is not sterile or not acceptable in certain cultures.

Population control should be the first starting point.

Maternal death is the largest problem in World Health.

Friedman then Philpott in Salisbury (Zimbabwe) started this idea that it was feasible to train midwives with a partogram. Technology of doing studies should be helpful in improving random controlled trials.

International Primary Care Computing
G.M. Hayes and N. Robinson (Editors)
Elsevier Science Publishers B.V. (North-Holland)
© IMIA, 1991

8.1   DEMOGRAPHY AND IT

Population Classifications

Brian Jarman

Department of General Practice,St Mary's Hospital Medical School, Lisson Grove
Health Centre,London, NW8 8EG, 0(7)1-723 7169

Introduction

There is a vast volume of information available regarding the characteristics of the
population of the UK, both as individuals and as groups which can, if needed, be produced
and plotted geographically. It is possible, for instance, to study the geographical variation
of social factors, health status and the provision of service of various types. It is a wide subject
and I will only try to discuss in detail two topics - a) the data available at ward and district
level, and b) some of the practical problems associated with collecting ward data.

There is so much data available that it is at times difficult to digest all that there is. It is
necessary to be selective and use only that which is most relevant and useful. The plotting
of coloured maps of selected data can be very helpful as it enables people to absorb a lot
of information painlessly. It can help us to proceed along the path from data to information
to knowledge to action.

It is perhaps the last of these concepts - action - that is the most difficult to achieve. The
preceding steps are however essential if the action is to be rational ie based on reason. This
involves drawing conclusions from facts, information, knowledge and evidence and then
deciding the best course of action.

Why are population classifications and geographical data needed?

I would suggest that some important matters for which population classifications and
geographical data analysis are useful are:

- Analysis of social and health conditions
- Planning of local services
- Resource allocations from regions and districts to general practices
- Improving health care services and monitoring results

What data are available?

The following are some of the data that can be of use:

- Social and health status data about people in different groups and areas

- Health and other services provision data for these groups and areas

- Changes of these factors with time and geography.

For example, our Department has produced information for regions, districts, general practices, social services departments etc at electoral ward and at DHA level which includes the following standard package (which is being updated):

Health and Social Data Available at Ward Level

I. Population:
Disaggregated by 5 year age bands, sex and marital status for 1981

II. Composite Indices of Socio-Economic Deprivation:
1. UPA8 score/Jarman score and associated variables: namely, the percentage of all residents who are (i) pensioners living alone (ii) children under 5 (iii) lone parents (iv) unskilled (SEG11) (v) unemployed and seeking work or temporarily sick within the economically active age group (vi) living in overcrowded households (1 person/room) (vii) have changed address over the past year (viii) in households headed by a person born in the New Commonwealth or Pakistan.

2. Townsend deprivation score and associated variables: namely, the percentage of (i) economically active residents (aged 16- 59/64) who are unemployed (ii) households with no car (iii) households which are not owner occupied (iv) households which are overcrowded.

3. Department of Environment (DoE) Social, Economic, Housing and Basic Indices and associated variables namely, the percentage of residents who are (i) unemployed (aged 16-75 +) (ii) in households headed by a person born in the New Commonwealth or Pakistan (same as Jarman variable above); and the percentage of households (iii) in permanent buildings which are overcrowded (iv) which are single parent households (v) which lack basic amenities (vi) which contain one pensioner living alone.

4. Scottish Deprivation Index/Vera Carstairs Index and associated variables: namely, the percentage of residents who are (i) living in households with more than 1 person/room (same as Jarman variable above) (ii) in households where the head of household is in Social Class IV or V (iii) economically active males seeking work (iv) with no car.

III. Other Social Variables expressed as percentages:

    1. Unemployed males aged 16-64

    2. Unemployed females aged 16-59

    3. Permanently sick residents as a % of Economically active residents.

    4. Permanently sick residents as a % of All residents

    5. Temporarily sick residents as a % of Economically active residents

    6. Temporarily sick residents as a % of All residents

    7. Percentage of 17 year olds not in full time education

    8. Density of population 1981

    9. Percentage residents in Social classes I, II, IIIM IIIN, IV and V

    10. Socio-Economic Groups 1-17

IV Health Data

    1. Deaths: 1981 SMRs A, K and full age range 1981-85 average SMRs A, K and full age range.

    2. Births: 1981 Births disaggregated by sex. Livebirth and Stillbirths. Infant Mortality rate. % low-birth weight (–g) babies.

Health and Social Data Available at District Level

Demographic data
Total population, population under 75, and %s in 5 year age/sex groups

Health data

Infant & Perinatal mortality rates various years

Standardised mortality ratios (SMRs) for various years

Standardised mortality ratios up to ages 65, 75 & 85

SMR by ICD group weighted by ICD group hospital utilisation (used for the 1976 Resource Allocation Working Party - RAWP- formula)

SMR by ICD group, average for 1982 to 1987 (plus average number district deaths in each ICD group)

Actual & expected deaths, full age range and to age 75

Immunisation uptakes in 1985, children born 1983, DHSS estimates

Social data

Underprivileged area (UPA) score and component variables 1981 (means & SDs for England)

Range of social data from 1981 census & several deprivation indices (72 variables in all)

Health and health service provision

Nursing home data

General practitioners % aged 65 +

General practitioner average list size (FPC and OPCS population per GP)

Community health service expenditure data

Data regarding hospital consultants & junior doctors

Expected expenditure on hospital services 1993/94 from Regional Strategic Plans

Percentage expenditure change 1983/4 to 1993/4 from Regional Strategic Plans

Standardised bed availability score

Bed availability score (weighted mean of beds/1000 resident population of the central district weighted x 2, with adjacent districts weighted x1)

Available beds/1000 resident population

Unused beds availability score

Actual deaths and discharges of district resident population

Predicted deaths and discharges of district resident population, various models.

Ratio of expected deaths and discharges old RAWP & RAWP review models to White Paper model

As above for average beds used daily (1983 and 1985)

Standardised values for above models (ratio actual D&D/ABUD to expected values by model x100)

Actual deaths and discharges & average beds used daily for patients treated in each district 1983/5

From this, treatment costs calculated from average costs/case and 7 specialty group costs/case

Standardised D&D/ABUD ratios (age/sex/marital status expected values) for specialty groups

Average waiting list times in weeks for different age-groups

Practical Issues

Population accuracy
For resource allocation it is essential that the population base used for calculations of resources is the same as that which is relevant to the use of those resources in practice. For instance, sub-regional district hospital allocations are usually based on the OPCS population estimates of resident populations of a district. These can be very different from the actual populations treated in areas where there is high population mobility, homelessness etc. In inner city areas the FHSA general practitioner list sizes are 30% higher than the OPCS population estimates. Some of this is as a result of under-enumeration of the census (4% in inner London), some due to general practitioners' list 'inflation' and some due to the fact that the address given by the patient when they are admitted to hospital (and hence the address used for the hospital records) is often different from the address which would be taken at the time of enumeration of the census.

This will continue to be very important after April 1991 when the NHS Review is implemented and hospital resources are allocated to resident populations. We found that 90% of the variance of hospital usage could be explained by variations in population size alone (ie health and social factors were less powerful explanatory variables). A 5% discrepancy between the population measure used for resource allocation and the actual population which is treated in a district would result in a 5% discrepancy in the correct resource allocation. The community charge registers will give a population data base which may not accurately reflect actual service usage in an area and hence may be inaccurate.

Confidentiality

The full computerisation of the general practitioner patient registration system at the NHS Central Register (covering about 98% of the ordinarily resident population) may make this the most accurate and relevant population register that we have. There are of course confidentiality problems here and these have yet to be resolved fully. The lists which general practitioners have of their patients have considerable potential use for the NHS (and others) for planning and providing services to a defined population. However these data should only be used for the purposes for which they were provided and a small but significant proportion of patients do not wish any of their personal details to go beyond their general practitioner.

Obtaining the data

This can be a major problem. A lot of data are not available for what are said to be confidentiality reasons. The UK is in a better position than many European countries in this respect, e.g. in Germany there is much less information regarding variations in death rates and less local information about health care provision. Different countries have different ideas about what is confidential and one wonders at times whether confidentiality is main reason for data non-availability.

Ward data problems
Analysis of ward data linking health and social conditions has a number of pitfalls:
> The boundary changes for 20% - 30% of wards since 1981. To analyse the 3.6 million deaths from 1981 to 1985 by ward we will have to use a 1981 frozen post-code directory to put the data to 1981 boundaries.

> The need for a look-up table to go from ward social data to ward vital statistics (deaths etc) data. This can be difficult to obtain but is essential.

> The problems with post-coded data.

> These arise because the grid reference of a post-code is the point of the 100m national grid reference which is the nearest to the South West of the area of streets etc covered by the post-code. Post-coding is accurate to 100 metres, and less so if the post-code directory is not up-to-date. We have found, in London, errors of about 12% in post-coding addresses to electoral wards and about 50% errors in post-coding to Enumeration Districts.

Enumeration Districts (EDs)
These are the small areas covered by an enumerator at the time of the census. They cover about 150 families, 450 people. There are problems in locating addresses to EDs, as mentioned, and also in plotting the EDs as there are 110,000 of them in England and Wales.

'Cut-off' problems for deciding on service provision

If action is to be taken eg at ward level using measures of social deprivation, then there will be "hidden areas of deprivation" which will not be recognised if the areas are considered on a ward basis and there are substantial parts of the wards which are not deprived and parts of other wards which are deprived (by whatever measure is used). The best way of dealing with this is to examine the ED data which applies to variations within a ward.

However, wards are more stable in their characteristics than EDs and their average population is about 5300. It is therefore probably best to identify deprivation nationally on a ward basis but to be able to study locally, using ED data and local knowledge, the variations within wards where they are significant.

Inconsistencies in data collection

In Scotland the ethnic and overcrowding variables were recorded differently in 1981 from the way they were recorded in England, Wales and Northern Ireland. It has been necessary to make adjustments to allow for these differences in Scotland in order to make the data comparable with the rest of the UK. In Northern Ireland there was some under-recording of the census in some areas.

If in Wales the index used to measure deprivation is altered, then there will appear to be a discrepancy along the Wales/England border - probably with Welsh wards appearing to have higher scores than their neighbours in England.

What to do with resources

We are just beginning to be able to distribute our resources more appropriately in health care on a small area basis. Not only do we have to decide where the needs are greatest, we also have the whole debate regarding what is the best action to take. It is difficult to demonstrate that any health care services have an effect in reducing overall mortality rates in an area. In addition to health services, housing and education are generally considered to be important for improving the quality of people's lives. So also is the efficient use of social security payments to those who are poor or disabled. We have work to do in establishing the correct balance between these services and learn how to target them in order to make the best use of finite resources.

International Primary Care Computing
G.M. Hayes and N. Robinson (Editors)
Elsevier Science Publishers B.V. (North-Holland)
© IMIA, 1991

8.2 Seminar Report: Demography and IT

Chairman :Dr G. Dove, North End Medical Centre 211 North End Road London W14 9WT UK

Presenter :Prof. B.Jarman, Lisson Grove Health Centre Gateforth Street London NW8 8EG UK

Discussant: Dr R. Turner, Hull Health Authority Victoria House Park Street Hull HU2 8TD UK,

Rapporteur: Dr Neill Jones, Marsden Road Health Centre Marsden Road South Shields SR6 7PN. UK

Demography and IT

Whatever horizons of demography were anticipated by the audience of twelve present at this seminar, it was soon apparent that Prof. Brian Jarman intended to confine a subject with so indefinite a title to his own brief, which was how the British National Health Service could respond to areas of deprivation of one sort or another, in so far as such areas could be determined.

He had had an interest in this problem for the last decade and come to the conclusion that evidence for an enquiry of this type could best be calculated from analysis of information collected for the 1981 British National Census. Once allowed permission into this Government domain, he has by a complex number crunching exercise now possible by the advance in IT, determined parameters for such a study. His work had had the objective of weighing factors by giving them numbers depicting differing values of vulnerability, deprivation and/or health needs, and defining such needs on a community based grid. Thus deprived areas would be getting a greater share of the cake than others.

The Standard Mortality Rate in each Ward provided an initial indicator, when if examined by age, differing needs were quickly identified, e.g. under 65, and under 75 groups. The latter showed increased resources wanted in areas preferred by the elderly.

By elaborating his coded system, derived from weighting a wide range of social, family, and medical variables, he defined his measure - the UPA Score. The application of this score, appropriate to what funds were available (a figure of 160 being accepted as critical) enable a differential to be established.

Based on a demographic grid to define individual units, a more accurate distribution of resources to them was possible. These units are made up by the amalgamation of a number of adjacent Post Codes districts, (a useful although not accurate border for such a unit - a unit to be known as a Ward - the British Isles thus geographically broken up into a number of such Wards). By definition a Ward should contain 5,000 persons. The average UPA of such a Ward would then activate increased expenditure if over the 160 mark.

Professor Jarman conceded that as the 1981 Census was ten years out of date, many of the results he had obtained were inconsistent with the times. To update such a model he suggested that deprived individuals or families could be pinpointed more accurately both in position and need, by their General Practitioner undertaking the task himself. First the GP would pinpoint the front door of the applicant by use of the National Grid reference map, then apply the Jarman Code to substantiate each claim.

This reverse feedback to the FPCs would enable an updated accurate records system of real deprivation to be centralised and directed the resources to where they are actually now needed.

Dr Turner questioned whether Post Codes had any value, since they are proved to be 55% inaccurate. He raised the issue as to whether such informative intelligence impinged on patient/doctor confidentiality, especially if the Area Health Councils and FPCs were to be amalgamated in the future (this amalgamation was considered to be unlikely).

The overall opinion was that any such action would initiate the possibility of a "Big Brother" intrusion into the individual life circumstances of the vulnerable person, while at the same time would give sensitive information to a wide range of linked bureaucratic bodies.

The creation of the Jarman Index, although seen to have inherent social and political problems in its implementation, was considered a useful index as a spring board for work in defining areas of deprivation, analogous in some extent to Read Coding as a means of identifying medical audit with which it could be used in conjunction.
One result might be that vulnerable individuals, defined as deprived, might find it easier to get on GPs' lists; another, that a wider use of such an accurate system will contribute to an assortment of epidemiological studies in all fields of medicine, social progress and examination for industrial or geographically based illnesses.

International Primary Care Computing
G.M. Hayes and N. Robinson (Editors)
Elsevier Science Publishers B.V. (North-Holland)
© IMIA, 1991

9   MEDICAL RECORDS

9.1   Primary Care Medical Records:

A Proposed Structure to Encourage their Use

Sheila Warshawsky

Division of Health in the Community, Ben-Gurion University of the Negev, Beersheva, Israel.

It is well established that the medical record of today is the principal instrument for ensuring continuity of care. If properly organised, the medical record can serve as an information system to document the medical history of the patient as well as a data base for patient and clinic management, epidemiologic studies and medical research.

Several computerized medical records systems have been developed to achieve this comprehensive function. Most of these systems rely on the use of data-entry forms by the professional, followed by data entry via data-entry clerks. Drawbacks of this type of system include illegibility of the coded forms causing recording errors, time lag from patient encounter to data entry and in entering lab results, inaccessibility of the complete patient record a the time of patient/physician encounter, and added cost of data-entry clerks.

Medical record systems that are based on direct entry by the user, whether that may be the physician, the nurse, the medical secretary, the laboratory technician, or the clinic pharmacist can eliminate these drawbacks while giving the user the added benefit of having the complete records available instantaneously in a clear, legible, organized format. Computerized medical records systems should be implemented in primary care clinics all over the world and these systems, in order to achieve their optimum, should be constructed to allow for the user to use the system for direct documentation as well as for information retrieval. However, systems should be adapted to specific geographic locations and to the specific abilities of the user. The system should allow for the creation of one computerized medical record for each member of the population.

The paramount goal of primary care computerized medical records must be to get them into use. This can only be done by making the systems match the sites - no universal system with a fixed medical content can work. A basic system that can be adapted to the site may be the answer. In general the basic goals of a computerized medical record for use in a primary care clinic should be:

- 1. To computerize the medical record based on the Problem Oriented Record i.e that imitates how a physician routinely works

The medical content of the computerized medical record is best organized according to the Problem Oriented Record - an acknowledged method of record keeping developed by Larry Weed [1]. The Problem Oriented Record consists of a clinical data base, problem list(s), problem oriented plans and problem oriented progress notes for documentation of an encounter. Progress notes follow the format of subjective, objective, assessment, plan (SOAP). Patient data can be organized in several ways such as summary sheets, previous encounters, graphic displays. The system should allow for documentation of encounters, laboratory and special tests results, routine examinations, demographic and family history, and any other specific requirements of the location. In parallel with this documentation, the system should allow for creation of a data base of the population.

- 2. To allow for direct data entry by the physician so that the physician has online access to the complete patient record during an encounter;

- 3. To create a system that is easy to use and fast;

- 4. To produce a system where the doctor would receive some benefits that would help him in his administrative tasks such as automatic printing of prescriptions, lab requests, and referrals;

- 5. To allow for the use of all the information collected in the data base for community health monitoring, reporting, and looking for trends in the health of our population.

- 6. To produce a system that can be used by all of the clinic staff;

- 7. To allow for adaptation for use by different members of the clinic staff, in different parts of the world, according to their specific requirement.

In other words, the system has to be both usable and utilitarian so that the physician and the staff will use it.
How can such a system be usable i.e. how to make direct entry a pleasure, not a chore - and how can such a system be utilitarian -i.e. how to organize the patient and clinic records so that all the information is accessible?

The keys to such a system are:

1. organization of the medical content
2. coded help menus to facilitate direct data entry and information retrieval.

How can the Medical Content be Organized?

The medical content has to be organized to facilitate documentation using direct entry. Problems and diseases endemic and prevalent to a region can be grouped into categories according to common signs and symptoms. Each category has its own set of progress notes (SOAP) with corresponding coded help menus. Each coded help menu should appear on the screen with its SOAP section so that there is no need to remember the code or to look for them on another screen or window.

How are Coded Help Menus Constructed?

The essence is that this is a team effort where lists of important points are extracted from relevant algorithms for each category of problems. These points are organized into coded help menus that match the divisions of the progress notes. Organizing the medical content into categories of problems allows for the construction of workable grouping for each category rather than having long data dictionaries covering wider areas.

Coded help menus not only facilitate data entry but also serve as reminders for patient management. The coded help menus not only provide a usable way to document but also allow for easy information retrieval since most entry is via codes - that is, the utility factor is high.

Use of a computer by a physician during a patient encounter had been thought an impossibility because of:

1. the characteristics of medical science,
2. the nature of a physician's thinking,
3. the personal quality of the physician/patient encounter
4. and the newness of medical computing in primary care.

A direct-entry computerized medical record system CLINIC [2] based on organizing medical content according to categories of problems and utilizing algorithm based help menus has been in use in a primary care clinic in Yerucham, Israel. The CLINIC project shows that physicians will use a computer during a patient encounter if they feel that the system has a benefit and resembles the medical record. The coded help menus combined with the design of the system in categories of problems facilitates use of the computer. This way of thinking can naturally be extended to design screens for any type of clinic tasks. It can be as simple as required by the user or as sophisticated as needed. This type of system has the potential to be applied any place in the world and to be used to both document information and make that information available in meaningful, easily accessible format.

References

1. Weed LL. Medical records that guide and teach. NEJM 1968; 278: 593-652.
2. Warshawsky S, Urkin J, Dagan O, Margolis C, Goldfarb D, Abusallah M, Elkiany A. In: Proceedings HC 90--Current Perspectives in Health Computing; British Computer Society, 1990; pp. 262-266.

International Primary Care Computing
G.M. Hayes and N. Robinson (Editors)
Elsevier Science Publishers B.V. (North-Holland)
© IMIA, 1991

9.2   Direct Data Entry by Medical Personnel

Sheila Warshawsky, Jacob Urkin, Oded Dagan, Carmi Z. Margolis, Dani Goldfarb,
Mouhammed Abusallah, Asher Elkiany.

Faculty of Health Sciences,Ben Gurion University of the Negev, Beersheva, Israel.

The medical record of today serves as documentation of the patient medical history as well as a source for medical data bases. This paper reports on the CLINIC system that computerizes the medical record and allows for direct data-entry by the medical personnel during an encounter via a system based on categories of problems and complaints with common signs and symptoms. The CLINIC system is currently being used in a primary care clinic.

Introduction

The medical record is commonly accepted today as the principal instrument for ensuring continuity of care.[1] If properly organized, the medical record can serve as an information system to document the medical history of the patient as well as a data base for patient and clinic management, epidemiologic studies and medical research. Several computerized medical records systems have been developed to achieve this comprehensive function [1-3]. Most of these systems rely on the use of data-entry forms by the professional, followed by data entry via data-entry clerks. Draw-backs of this type of system include illegibility of the coded forms causing recording errors, time lag from patient encounter to data entry and in entering lab results, inaccessibility of the complete patient record at the time of patient/physician encounter, and added cost of data-entry clerks [2,3].

The CLINIC computerized medical record system eliminates these drawbacks and maximizes the potential of a computerized medical record system by:

1. allowing for direct data entry by the physician during a patient encounter using coded help menus;
2. allowing for direct access by the physician to the complete medical record of the patient during an encounter;
3. allowing for documentation of the encounter according to the Problem Oriented Record (POR) and organized using the format of subjective, objective, assessment, plan (SOAP).[4]
4. providing for easy retrieval in report form of the information in the resulting data base.

The key to the successful implementation of this direct-entry system is the structure of the system which incorporates the following features:

1. CLINIC is organized according to categories of problems and diseases having common signs and symptoms;
2. Each category of problems has specific coded help menus for each section of the POR;

136

3. The coded help menus for each problem are algorithm based.[5] A team of physicians authored and organized the medical content of the screens;

4. Each coded help menu appears on the screen with its corresponding section. There is no need to remember the codes or to look for them on another screen.

Background

The CLINIC Computerized Medical Record System was developed at Ben Gurion University, Israel for use in community primary care clinics. The system is currently being run as a pilot study in the primary care clinic in the desert town of Yeruham. The clinic, serving a population of 6,000 of mainly lower socio-economic status, is divided into a pediatric unit and an adult unit, each with two physicians and a nurse. Patients are not assigned to a particular physician. Prior to computerizing the clinic, medical information was kept as handwritten notes in folders. Lab, x-ray, consultation notes and test results were often placed in the folders separately. Reviewing a patient record was tedious and the record was often incomplete and illegible. A general data base from these records was unavailable. The CLINIC system has been in use for 2 1/2 years by 6 different physicians as well as two nurses and a medical secretary. Help menus exist for 15 categories of common primary care problems. 20,000 encounters have been documented. One hundred reports have been generated.

Equipment

The program is currently run on a Motorola 6350 mini-computer under Unix with 6 terminals located in the offices of the physician, medical secretary and nurse. Each has a printer. There is another terminal at the University for software development, linked to Yeruham by a modem. Backup is done weekly on a magnetic tape and monthly in hardcopy. The system is currently being transferred to a Digital Equipment Corporation VAX minicomputer.

Software

The CLINIC system is based on an application generator written in MUMPS. Data entry is via numbered codes to the field from the help menu which is automatically displayed on the bottom of each screen. The user touch-types the appropriate number on the keypad. The system also allows free text input via direct typing in the field. Multiple codes can be entered in one field, thus chaining words and descriptors. Coded data and free text can be intermingled in the same field. Depending on the type of encounter CLINIC provides several ways of documentation:

1. A short entry screen with a corresponding coded help menu on the same screen for a common, uncomplicated problem;

2. A series of SOAP subdivision screens for the more extensive documentation of an acute problem. Every screen has a

corresponding coded help menu developed from clinical algorithms for that particular category of problems;

3. Flowsheets for the followup of chronic problems;

4. Extensive checklists for routine examinations.

In addition to documenting an encounter, CLINIC provides coded screens for the automatic generation of the following forms resulting from an encounter: prescriptions, lab test requests, referral letters, work permits, and health permits. Test results are also entered using appropriate coded screens.

CLINIC allows for the organization of patient data in several ways such as summary sheets, encounters, flow sheets according to time, and graphic displays superimposed over standardized graphs. The summary sheets available for each patient include demographic data, problem list, medications, recent encounters and hospitalizations, allergies, well-baby care, chronic diseases and medications, lab results, routine physical check list, family history, followups and reminders as to routine vaccinations and tests. A report generator allows the user to retrieve information from the data base of the clinic population.

Physician Use of Computer During an Encounter

Following is a breakdown of a routine patient encounter:

1. The physician logs in according to a password;

2. The patient's record is located by name or identification number;

3. A summary screen automatically is displayed;

4. The physician reviews past encounters and additional summary

screens as needed;

5. Discussion between physician and patient about reason for visit;

6. Physical examination;

7. Physician documents encounter. Data are entered using free- text or coded numbers from the help menu. In most cases the physician uses the terminal intermittently during the encounter, in the "conversational" encounter strategy.[6]

8. Computer prints out necessary forms such as prescriptions.

Implementation
Information from the written record was entered into CLINIC by a senior medical student. To date some 20,000 encounters have been documented with an average increase in the length of an encounter to be about 2 minutes (8-10 min). However, while documentation by handwritten notes is faster, the use of CLINIC seems to encourage the gathering of more explicit information due to the "suggestions" in the help menus. Time is saved during other routine office procedures by eliminating the need to physically locate the written record for the visit and for entering test results. Some 100 reports have been generated by the users of CLINIC for research teaching and service, such as locating patients during a 1988 chicken

pox epidemic, results of 1200 throat cultures in 1988-89, frequency of complaints and diagnoses in the pediatric unit, medication use in the clinic, frequency of visits to the clinic in the first year of life by month and sex.

Physicians using the computer feel that it eases their work load and organizes the medical record in such a way that the information contained within is accessible. The coded help menus combined with the design of the system in categories of problems facilitates use of the computer. Time was needed to adjust to the system, but each new user adapted quickly. There was no harm to the communication between the patient and the physician. The program was particularly successful when used for a short time by an immigrant doctor with poor written language ability.

Use of a computer by a physician during a patient encounter had been thought an impossibility because of the characteristics of medical science, the nature of a physician's thinking, the personal quality of the physician/patient encounter and the newness of medical computing in primary care.[1] The CLINIC project shows that physicians will use a computer during a patient encounter if they feel that the system has a benefit. With CLINIC, the physician gets organized patient records, easy access to the information within these records and the ability to easily document. Using the computer does not upset clinic procedures. Both the user and the patient were quickly at ease and felt a part of the modern world. CLINIC's success is undoubtedly due to the uniqueness of the system design - problems and diseases with common complaints and symptoms organized into categories with corresponding algorithm-based help menus specific for each category.

References

1. Barnett GO. The application of computer based-medical record systems in ambulatory practice. NEJM 1984; 25:1643-1650.

2. Dambro MR, Weiss BD, McClure CL, Vuturo AR. An unsuccessful experience with computerized medical records in an academic center. J Med Ed 1988; 63:617-623.

3. McDonald CJ, Tierney WM. Computer-stored medical records: their future role in medical practice. JAMA 1988; 23:3433-3440.

4. Weed LL. Medical records that guide and teach. NEJM 1968; 278: 593-562.

5. Margolis CZ. Solving Common Pediatric Problem: An Algorithm Approach. New York, The Solomon Press, 1988.

6. Brownbridge G, Evans A, Wall T. Effect of computer use in the consultation on the delivery of care. BMJ 1985; 639-642.

International Primary Care Computing
G.M. Hayes and N. Robinson (Editors)
Elsevier Science Publishers B.V. (North-Holland)
© IMIA, 1991

9.3 Medical Records - Notes by Rapporteur

Chairman :Dr Alan Rector, Medical Informatics Group Dept. of Computer Science Manchester University Oxford Road Manchester M13 9PL UK

Presenter :Mrs Sheila Warshawsky, Faculty of Health Sciences Ben Gurion University of the Negev Beersheva Israel.

Discussant: Dr Stuart Foote, Heretaunga Medical Centre 306 West Lyndon Road Hastings New Zealand

Rapporteur: Dr John Williams, 1 Woodruff Avenue Guildford Surrey GU1 1XS UK

Chairman's Opening Comments

The Chairman having introduced and welcomed all participants
opened the session by stating that high quality medical records were obviously essential. In a sense everything started from the medical record. He felt that ideally computer systems should be built from the bottom upwards. That meant finding out what doctors really needed from computers to help them with their work. In his experience this was no easy task as even things that seemed simple conceptually often turned out to be complex when put into practice.

Dr Warshawsky presented her paper entitled "Direct Data Entry by
Medical Personnel". She maintained that the Medical Record had to act as documentation of the patient's medical history as well as a source for medical databases. She was critical of the written record as being difficult to follow. Even when well organised it was only capable of linear (eg chronological) structure. Far more useful and complex structure could be achieved by using the Problem Oriented Record structure on computer.

It was highly desirable that data should be entered directly by
the health professional at the time of the encounter, and that data should only need to be entered once to be available to all who might wish to retrieve it. Some computer systems depended on health professionals using encounter (data entry) forms with clerical staff later transcribing the information from these forms to computer. Such systems were subject to problems:

  1) Illegible forms led to transcription errors

  2) There was a time lag between encounter and data entry to computer

  3) Entering of lab results could become delayed

  4) The health professional did not have access to the complete patient
     record when it would be most useful - at the time of the encounter

  5) Added cost of data entry clerks

She contrasted this with her experience of direct data entry using the "Clinic" system described in her paper:

1) The doctor had the whole record available at every encounter

2) The record was well organised, and data easily retrieved

3) The record was legible and easy to follow

4) Single data entry occurred at the time of consultation leading to greater accuracy, saving of time and money (cost of clerical staff)

5) The record was accessible to all

6) It was useful for training purposes, and for assessment during training

7) It was easy to retrieve information from the database in report form.

The "Clinic" system was based on the Problem Oriented Record.

It was a clinical database that incorporated problem lists, problem oriented plans, and problem oriented progress notes (SOAP) -

Subjective
Objective
Assessment
Plan

She found that eighty five per cent of patients presented with one or more of seven common problems. Virtually all presentations could be covered with a list of one hundred problems which in turn could be grouped into fifteen categories (containing problems and diseases sharing common signs and symptoms). Having established these categories a list of relevant points had been made for each one based on algorithms, and literature, peer, and specialist review. Then using this information help menus had been designed for every SOAP division for each category. These help menus could easily be called up, and coded entries with or without free text could be typed in at the time of the encounter, using these menus as prompts. The system had been in use for two and a half years by six different physicians and two nurses. On average the length of an encounter had increased by about two minutes (from eight to ten minutes). Physicians felt that the system had eased their workload and made information more accessible, although time had been needed to adjust to the system.

Doctor/patient communication had not been adversely affected.

Dr Foote felt that the Medical record was an essential aid to the doctor in delivering patient care. It might be needed to defend the doctor's actions. It should be capable of supporting audit both of the individual doctor and collectively. There was a clear connection between good records and quality of care although the former did not guarantee the latter. It was important to remember that the doctor's prime purpose was not to accumulate data but to assess patients and offer them appropriate treatment.

There were a number of important trends affecting Primary care.

1) Reduction of inpatient care with more responsibility put on to the GP for more complex mixes of problems.

2) Need for better management in dimension of time - e.g. call/recall facilities for follow-up.

3) Need to identify groups with particular requirements, and need for method(s) of delivering care to these patients.

4) Need for knowledge assistance - expert systems integrated with medical records.

5) Need for increased accountability, quality assurance due to greater expectations both of individuals and of corporate entities providing care - "Cost Effectiveness".

6) Need for better continuity of care. Medical record should be as mobile as the patient.

The paper record currently in use was simply not capable of meeting all these challenges. At best it acted as an aide memoire for the doctor actually making the note and did not even do that particularly well. Computers had the potential to fulfill all these needs. It would be necessary clearly to define the problems and objectives of computerised medical records.

A number of questions were posed:

1) Why should uptake of computers be so low in Primary care

2) What could be done to promote better uptake

3) In what directions should R & D be heading - can they solve problems relating to the interface with doctor and with patient? Would systems be able to cope with all problems presented how ever complex and unexpected they might be. Would they be able to produce the information needed by individual doctors, the profession as a whole, and politicians. Would such systems be acceptable to doctors and patients?

General Discussion

A lively discussion followed and a number of points were registered:

1) The medical record should not be confused with the consultation.

2) The medical record is more than just clinical notes. It also includes letters, forms and results.

3) The purpose of the medical record needs to be clearly defined.

4) When thinking about the format of a computerised medical record we should not restrict our imagination by always relating back to existing paper records.

5) The structure of computerised medical records need not necessarily be based on SOAP.

6) When assessing potential systems it is necessary not just to check their ability to cope with common problems but also their flexibility when faced with unusual/unforeseen events.

7) In order to get maximum benefit from computerised records it will be necessary to eliminate paper records.

8) For maximum efficiency it will be essential to get related bodies (eg Hospitals, Insurance companies, Family Practitioner Committees) to tailor their systems to make exchange of information as easy as possible (e.g. design of forms, method of data exchange).

9) The general need for standardisation and agreed protocols was acknowledged.

10) The need for an adequate audit trail documenting all changes to the record is paramount especially if written records are to be abandoned.

11) There should be an agreed code of practice for "backing up" records. A "backup" should enable a complete recovery and not just cover selected files. At present there seems to be no general agreement about what constitutes a "backup" or how often it should be done. There should also be a means of ensuring that "backups" are technically successful before recovery from a disaster reveals failure.

12) There was probably a need for an interface faster than pen and paper, otherwise all doctors might have to acquire typing skills. Was the keyboard really best? This area had already been covered in Workshop 1 - Interfacing Doctors."

13) Direct data entry dictates the need to use the computer during consultations. It was suggested that many doctors view this as obtrusive to the doctor patient relationship. It seems that "doctors have the hang up and not patients". There is certainly a need for the doctor to become familiar with the system and to adapt consultation style to the computer's presence - a definite learning time. Thereafter the positive advantages of being able to share data validation and decision making with the patient become more obvious. Patients seem to expect professionals to use modern technology. It should not be forgotten that paper records can be very obtrusive. The use of video might help to persuade doctors who have any doubts in this area.

14) A more valid objection to using the computer during the consultation might be that many systems currently available simply do not perform the tasks that doctors really need.

15) Computer generated referral letters were viewed as a mixed blessing. Some consultants apparently welcome the extra information conveyed to them while others object to the loss of a proper "letter". The distinction was made between "form" and "letter". It might be necessary to generate both when making a referral, to enhance the quality of data transmitted and yet retain the personal touch.

16) It was claimed that direct data entry on to a computer without the need to maintain written records led to a fall in the total net time required to maintain medical records throughout the Practice, although in some areas the amount of time needed obviously rose. Some members were unhappy about the entry of other information

(e.g. letters). It would take time to select the data needing input, and then actually to enter it.

17) The advantages of having a computerised medical record could be grouped under two headings:

- Ease of seeing patient

- Ease of running the Practice

Clarity of information and ease of retrieval were highlighted as the most obvious benefits.

18) Reasons cited for reluctance on the part of doctors to computerise included the lack of any financial return, the financial outlay and absence of any commercial benefit, poor data capture facilities, and pressure of time. What was the point of spending time and energy structuring records if it was possible to "get away without doing it". In the UK political and financial pressures were the main driving force leading to consensus that computerisation was necessary part of survival.

Closing Comments

The Chairman briefly summarised by stating that there seemed to be consensus overlying some confusion. In his experience when attempting to establish what doctors really needed from their systems it often turned out that for every item wanted three more were actually needed, although some of these might already have been supplied elsewhere. In this Workshop there had clearly been a consensus in favour of fully computerised medical records and abandonment of the written record.

Addendum: Important Features of the Computerised Medical Record

This did not form part of the workshop - but the need to define the purpose / problems / properties of the MR was voiced on several occasions. Below are some of the salient points raised both in the papers presented and during the workshop.

1) Information system documenting patient's medical history

2) Database for

patient management

clinic management

epidemiological studies

medical research

3) Essential aid to doctor in delivering patient care

a) Over a period of time (eg call / recall)

    b) In identifying populations of patients

    c) In identifying needs of groups of patients

    d) In assisting with delivery of care

4) Record to defend actions

5) Should be integrated with Practice administration

6) Should support audit - both individual and collective

7) Should be integrated with Knowledge Assistance (Expert systems). Linkage with management protocols

8) Should hold necessary data to support accountability / quality assurance / Cost Effectiveness - both for individuals and providers of resources

9) Should cater for patient mobility - continuity of care when patient moves

10) Orderly structure essential

11) Should support automatic checks eg for contra- indications, and to aid opportunistic care

12) Should support agreed protocols and standards

13) Should be supported by audit trail

14) Should be protected by adequate backup protocols

15) Should be secure

International Primary Care Computing
G.M. Hayes and N. Robinson (Editors)
Elsevier Science Publishers B.V. (North-Holland)
IMIA, 1991

10 SECURITY AND DATA PROTECTION

10.1 The Six Safety First Principles of Health Information Systems

Barry Barber

NHS Information Management Centre, 19 Calthorpe Road, Birmingham B15 1RP, England

The Scenario for Health Care in Europe

Clinicians and health care practitioners are only effective if they meet the needs of their patients and managers are only effective if they meet the needs of their organisations. Meeting patients' needs means knowing what they are, communicating them to the nearest decision maker and outwards as far as necessary to do something to enable the needs to be met. In this fashion the Health Care activities are driven by patients' needs. The patient will expect to share in the decisions about his care or that of his family and will further expect that there will be staff with the knowledge, skill, and ability to act on these decisions. Correspondingly, the totality of the needs of the organisation sets the agenda for the managers' activities. Some of these ideas were developed by Scholes, Abbot and Barber (1989).

Political issues and health care ethics will of necessity be part of the decision process. To this end patient self care and self assessment will be encouraged, so that the identification of health problems and home treatment can be supported. There is no doubt that there is an exploding information base that technology can make readily accessible to the majority of the population.

The following issues stand out for serious attention:

Increasingly Elderly Population requiring more Health Services
The statistical projections show increasing numbers of elderly individuals in the population of Europe. This population group places relatively heavy demands on the Health and Welfare Services.

The emphasis of the Health Services should be towards that of ensuring high standards in the quality of life with appropriate access to desired care. The UK Dept of Health Statistical Bulletin covering acute care during the period 1974-1985 showed an overall increase of 20% in the acute in-patients treated but this included an increase of 80% in those treated over 75 years old. Demographic change only accounted for half of this increase. In terms of the caring necessary to support individuals age may not be the key issue but rather the individual's mobility and mental capacity.

This trend has been accompanied by further confounding sociological factors: the changing role of women, particularly in their labour force participation and their availability as "family carers", and an increasingly mobile society. Thus an increasing proportion of the elderly live alone or in institutions resulting in a high, and increasing, need for various patterns of institutional and domiciliary care.

This pattern is typical of many developed countries around the world and it appears to be reasonably representative of the European Community as a whole. This three-way squeeze will put great pressure on the health care systems of Europe and the resources available to them. The economic and social implications of this population ageing are explored in a United Nations Report (1988) and Oggawa (1982) indicating that major changes in funding are to be expected when the expenditure on Health Care exceeds about 7%.

Increasing Ability to Provide Life-Saving and Life-Enhancing Services
Current medical knowledge allows much more effective interventions but it is necessary to find a balance between mortality compression and morbidity decompression. Significantly more operations are being undertaken and they are more complex in character. Developments in operative procedures and organ transplants are fuelling this increase. These increases are already substantially greater than would be expected from the age-specific changes in the population. It can be expected that the progress in medical knowledge and the adoption of new techniques in bio-engineering and bio-technology will accentuate these developments.

Increasing Expectations that Services will be Provided
The population of Europe are becoming more aware of the possibilities available to them in Health Care Services and know that services can be provided successfully to much older people than were thought practical previously. The over 65s are likely to increase from approximately 10% of the population currently to around 20% during the early part of the next century.

The "Old Elderly" (over 75s, or even more so the over 85s) can consume substantial resources as they are likely to require more resources for a given clinical problem and of course they are likely to return for subsequent care after successful treatment. The Health Care costs have been estimated as six times those of equivalent patients under 65 years old but the social service costs are estimated at around 26 times. Changes in social habits are, also, leading to greater numbers of single-adult households which leads to higher health care costs where there is no supportive home environment. This development may need to be complemented by the clustering of single-adult households to provide mutual support or the basis for efficient community support in "granny towns". The social structures of the EC have barely addressed the needs that will emerge even though the current boom in retirement homes hints at things to come.

For instance, despite considerable measures to improve the efficiency of the UK National Health Service, increasing manpower and increased real resources, there is a definite gap between the resources currently being made available for health care and the expectations of the population. The national statistics indicate the additional activity undertaken for the population but it does not match expectations as to the care that, not only can, but that should be made available. Decisions about who gets what Health Care are very difficult whether they are personal in respect of available financial resources or national in respect of what facilities can be built and staffed.

Reducing pool of individuals available to staff the Health Services
The population projections indicate a reduction in the numbers of individuals in the economically active age bands. This effect may well be modified by changing patterns of economic activity in individuals and within the economy as a whole but it requires action in broadly the same direction as that required by the ageing population. Currently, it seems that Europe has enough qualified medical staff but they are not necessarily appropriately distributed. The provision of sufficient nursing staff may be a much greater problem. It is important that proper steps should be taken to ensure that there should be adequate monitoring of the European supply of Health Care Professionals and steps taken to ensure that they can move easily around the EC to where their skills may be needed.

Need for Greater Education and Support for Patients/Customers
The patients, or customers for the Health Services, will need to be much more widely educated in the opportunities and limitations of the services that can be provided so that they can more readily make informed choices about their life styles and preferences.

Political constraints on the availability of funds to provide Health Services
Throughout Europe there are difficulties in securing more funds for Health Care Services from the national revenue. All governments are anxious to contain costs by improving efficiency in the delivery of care and additional sources of revenue are being sought. Insurance based systems are similarly vulnerable, since higher health expenditure leads to a higher cost of labour and a potential decrease in international competitiveness.

Trends in Medical Informatics: Increasing Activity

There is a sharply increasing volume of activity both within hospitals and within the community. Computing is becoming more clinical and closer to the process of providing patient care. From clinical word processing to clinical department computing with more imaging systems and more decision support systems all these developments are edging clinical systems into the safety critical systems area.

The computing systems and advanced scanning equipment already installed enable more and more data to be available on the condition of patients and more and more scans to be carried out. There are now computer terminals linked to the major systems capable of accessing a variety of different systems rather than being dedicated to one system. More systems function throughout the 24 hours and more systems are accessed from outside the institutional environment. The systems are much more extensive and handle a larger range of clinical databases.

Together with the increasing activity and range of system facilities, technical developments also affect the scene. The explosive increase in the number of very powerful micro computers with large, fast internal storage together with very substantial backing store and communications facilities offers opportunities for much more creative purposes than the word processing and handling small scale databases for which they are mostly used at the moment.

When they are made more convenient to use and are more conveniently linked with the main Health Care systems Health Service usage will grow exponentially before saturating at a very high level. Distributed databases with easy access, enquiry and presentational mechanisms will transform the process of handling and utilising large volumes of information. Similarly, multi-media facilities will transform the education and training markets and the processes of implementing systems.

In some cases this extends to capability in the area of Telemedicine as the search for administrative efficiency, manpower reductions and improved clinical support leads to the more effective exploitation of major centres of medical expertise. Networked systems and distributed data bases are developing to facilitate this trend. The advent of smart cards may lead to readable, universal, reliable medical records but complex procedures are required for handling the transfer of medical data.

The following pattern is emerging:

     1 More terminals and computers

     2 More types of system - especially clinical applications

     3 More systems functioning 24 hours a day

     4 More systems accessed from outside the institution

     5 More systems networked

     6 More systems using distributed databases

     7 Safety critical systems developments

This pattern is one of increasing activity and increasingly important activity.

Increasing and Uncritical Reliance on Health Systems

With the increasing volume of activity in Health Informatics there has developed an increasing reliance on Health Systems in the provision of Health Care. In the earlier phases of the development of Health Systems, they were very much an adjunct to manual systems and most staff were experienced in working without access to such systems. It was not surprising that, despite everyone's best endeavours, the systems sometimes failed to work, or indeed, produced wrong answers. Great efforts were made to ensure that the systems were available when needed and functioned correctly but no-one was surprised when the combinations of hardware and software then available failed to live up to expectations.

Over the intervening years the efforts to achieve 24 hour accurate and reliable operation have slowly produced results and the present generation of systems is much more satisfactory. However, the fact that errors are not very common does not mean that they do not, or cannot, occur. Instead, it means that the users are not often faced with non-operational systems and, hence, the need to proceed without their assistance nor are they checking the results provided by the computers to see that they are broadly sensible. Health Professionals are slowly getting accustomed to operational systems that can achieve a massive amount of work within a very short time scale so that any failure of the systems to function can mean that there can be no chance of handling the work manually within the necessary time scale if the systems fail.

This increasing, and increasingly uncritical, reliance on computer systems in Health Care will increase as more useful decision support and safety critical systems are developed and brought into routine use. It is, therefore, vital that the issues of Computer Security should be properly addressed. An examination of these issues within the context of the Single European Market has led to the conclusions described below about the safety and reliability requirements for the next generation of European Health Information Systems.

The Six Safety First Principles

The following six Safety Principles should form that future basis of all use of Health Care Informatics in Europe. These requirements, which have been accepted by the AIM Requirements Board as a whole, are set out in quite general terms in order that they may be seen apart from the computing technicalities and so that detailed work can be focussed appropriately rather than constrained too early by particular approaches to solving certain problems.

As with the Data Protection Principles embodied in the Council of Europe Convention "For the Protection of Individuals with Regard to Automatic Processing of Personal Data", it will take some time before the full implications of these principles become apparent. Nevertheless, it is important that they should be adopted as the basic reference standard for European Medical Informatics Systems as soon as possible. This is desirable from the point of view of all concerned with the use of informatics systems within the Health Care environment but it is of particular importance to the EC Informatics industry and to EC patients.

Safe Environment for Patients and Users
This is required to ensure that no one is damaged by the operation or non-operation of the systems. The Health Informatics environment must be safe for the users at all levels from

"Safety Critical Systems" downwards. The minimum requirement is that the systems must not harm patients, clients, operators of the system or the Health Care Professionals concerned with its use. Quality control, assessment and certification procedures must be devised to ensure that the systems function safely and fail in a safe fashion. There must be no iatrogenic disease arising from the use of Advanced Informatics Systems.

Secure Environment for Patients, Users and Others

This is required to ensure that information is not lost, corrupted or made available to unauthorised persons. The environment must be appropriately secure in terms of unauthorised access to, linkage of, alteration and destruction of Personal Data, Critical Reference Data, Health Care Knowledge within a Knowledge Base, Decision Support Software, Applications and Operating System Software or Hardware. The most stringent requirements of the Council of Europe Convention "For the Protection of Individuals with Regard to Automatic Processing of Personal Data" and the Regulations for Automated Medical Data Banks must be applied and be seen to be applied throughout the EC as well as other suitable requirements for non-Personal Data.

Convenient Environment for Users

This is required to ease the use of the systems and to reduce training needs. Health Informatics services will function most effectively within an environment in which such facilities are actively promoted and utilised. A number of Graphical User Interfaces (GUI) have been developed that provide very powerful environments in which users can handle the system functions with a minimum of detailed technical computing knowledge and training. In handling health records it is vital that the Computer Security systems should be as transparent as possible. Data that a Health Professional or his support staff are entitled to obtain should be readily and rapidly available but other data should be quite inaccessible.

Legally Satisfactory Environment Across Europe for Users and Suppliers

A clear specified and harmonious environment is required concerning the legal responsibilities for the development, marketing, maintenance and use and mis-use of systems. There are considerable areas of uncertainty regarding legal responsibility for various aspects of system performance, malfunction and usage. Harmonious legal, ethical and professional steps must be taken to ensure that responsibility for all aspects of the use of systems is unambiguously clarified and that these arrangements are compatible with other arrangements within the Health Care environment.

Product liability and the "duty of care" and the use or non-use of support systems are currently far from clear, even in the UK, let alone throughout the EC. This situation must be rectified swiftly if progress is to be made in developing a single market in advanced health care systems in Europe.

Legal Protection of Software Products
This is required in order to encourage the development and marketing of systems. If there is to be a vigorous market for Health Informatics Systems within Europe there must be adequate legal protection of software from unlicensed use as well as adequate quality assurance and testing of the products offered. The situation is analogous to the use of drugs where considerable effort is devoted to developing and testing safe drugs for particular medical conditions.

Multi-Lingual Systems
This is required in order to avoid errors from inadequate understanding of the local language and to facilitate the spread of systems throughout the EC. The variety of languages used within Europe makes it important that there should be convenient ways of implementing systems across linguistic boundaries without major customisation effort. This is another aspect of safety in that imperfectly understood medical terms in a foreign language might constitute a health hazard. Health Care Systems are so closely bound up with the precision that can only be obtained in the local language that considerable effort is required to ensure that European Systems can readily travel across national borders within the European Community. This will apply to the translation of codes, nomenclatures and classifications as well as to basic systems instruction manuals, knowledge embodied within the system and information output for the users.This process of translation, classification and coding requires central EC support if it is to function effectively and efficiently.

Conclusion

These six Safety First principles of Health Information Systems should be adopted as the European standard and considerable effort should be expended in ensuring that the systems and design implications of the principles are elucidated and put into practical effect.

Acknowledgements

This material has been taken directly from work undertaken for the European Commission's Advanced Informatics in Medicine (AIM) Requirements Board elaborated in a few places to make the context clearer.

References

Council of Europe Convention "For the Protection of Individuals with Regard to Automatic Processing of Personal Data" No 108, Stransbourg, 28/1/81 ISBN 92 871 0022 5 Explanatory Report on the Convention for the Protection of Individuals with Regard to Automatic Processing of Personal Data Stransbourg 1981

152

Council of Europe Regulations for Automated Medical Data Banks Recommendation No R (81) 1 Stransbourg 1981

Oggawa Population Ageing in Japan: Problems and Policy Issues in 21st Century, 1982, Nihon University, Tokyo

Scholes M, Abbott W & Barber B: Into the Next Millenium - Health Care and Information Management, MEDINFO 89, 8-13, North Holland Pub., Amsterdam, 1989

United Nations Organisation Economic and Social Implications of Population Ageing, 1988

International Primary Care Computing
G.M. Hayes and N. Robinson (Editors)
Elsevier Science Publishers B.V. (North-Holland)
© IMIA, 1991

10.2 Security and Data Protection: Report

Chairman :Dr Rory O'Moore, Dept. of Biochemistry St.James' Hospital James Street PO Box 580 Dublin 8

Presenter :Dr Barry Barber, NHS Information Management Centre 19 Calthorpe Road Edgbaston Birmingham B15 1RP UK

Discussant: Dr Nigel Harding,
Rapporteur: Dr Glyn Hayes, 3 Beech Avenue North, Worcester UK

A lively discussion followed the comprehensive introductory papers by Barry Barber [1] and Nigel Harding [2]. It was agreed very quickly that:

Firstly, the AIM Requirements Board developed the concepts of the Six Safety First Principles of Health Information systems [3-5,1] which should be adopted as "catch all" reference guidelines.

Secondly, the DHSS/FPS/BCS PHCSG Booklet Guidance on security standards for primary health care practitioners [6] should be recommended as the basic guidebook for computer security. The main reason for agreement was the perceived threat to good practice of data protection/confidentiality increasingly posed by rapid technological change. In particular, the areas of networking, advanced telecommunications and open systems interconnection, which are very relevant to future primary health care delivery. It was noted that the AIM Secretariat had sponsored a working conference on Data Protection and Legal Issues entitled "Handling Health Data in the Future in Europe -the Challenge of the New Technologies", 19-21 March 1990 in Brussels, and two volumes of Proceedings are being prepared.

The remainder of the discussion of WG1O is best summarised in the form of agreed urgent needs which emerged:

The need to develop a Reference Model for Healthcare Security/Confidentiality with particular reference to Primary Health care. This would allow various items of concern in Data Protection/Security which emerge in other Health Care fields to be mapped against the Model to determine relevance.

The need to agree definitions and terminology. At present "massive ambiguity" is the norm. For example, Data Security and Confidentiality are not synonymous. We must make our meaning clear, particularly in multi-lingual Europe.

The need for Audits, particularly in the form of testing and certification of systems and software. A probable role for some EEC body, such as CEN/CENELEC was envisaged.

The need to develop much greater awareness of the importance of confidentiality and data protection in both manual and computerised systems. There was general agreement in the group that standards at present were abysmal. We must be more aware of the rapid technological advances taking place and the security implications which ensue.

The need for educational initiatives to manage the impending technology 'leap'.

The need to define security of access to data. Who needs to know?

The need to define security of data transmission. Who is the data for, and why? In this context, the need to involve commercial partners in ALL aspects of data protection/security was stressed.

The need to define relative risks and determine prevention strategy. Procedures, such as, critical risk analysis and management methodology, CRAMM [8]. [Ref. B Davey in AIM Conference Handling Health Data in Europe in the Future. Proceedings 1990 AIM Office].

The need for professional codes of practice to be established for all health professionals involved in primary care.

The final agreed need was to re-establish the IMIA WG5 in primary care.

References

1. The Six Safety First Principles of Health Information Systems, Barber B, Jensen 0 A, Lamberts H, Roger F, de Schouwer P & Zollner H, in HC9O: Current Perspectives in Health Computing 1990 pub British Journal of Health Care Computing 1990 ISBN 0 948i98 09 5.

2. Security is a multidimensional, multilevel and growing problem. A fundamental building block (MEDIFACT) permits rational construction of reference models for a minimal risk strategy for ail health care systems. Nigel Harding & Angela Giles, Health Systems Coordination Office, 82 Lime Walk,Headington, Oxford OX3 7AY.

3. AIM Requirements Board, Impact Assessment and Forecasts of Information and Communications Technologies Applied to Health Care, Volumes I-IV, December 1989, ref XHI/F/A1O966C, AIM Secretariat, 61 Rue de Treves, Brussels.

4. Barber B, Jensen 0 A, Lamberts H, Roger F H, de Schouwer P & Zollner H, The Six Safety First Principles of Health Information Systems: A Programme of Implementation: Part 1 Safety and Security, Proc MIE-9O, Springer Verlag in press, 1990.

5. Barber B, Jensen 0 A, Lamberts H, Roger F H, de Schouwer P & Zoliner H, The Six Safety First Principles of Health Information Systems: A Programme of Implementation: Part 2 Convenience and Legal Issues, Proc MIE-9O, Springer Verlag in press, 1990.

6. "Guidance on Security Standards for Primary Health Care Practitioners, Department of Health and Primary Health Care Specialist Group.

7. EC AIM conference on Data Protection and Confidentiality in Health Informatics: 'Handling Health Data in Europe in the Future, 19-21 March 1990, Brussels, vols I and II in press.

8. CRAMM - A Guide for Management and User Guide, CCTA IT Security and Privacy Group, Riverwaik House, 157-161 Milibank, London SW1P 4RT.

International Primary Care Computing
G.M. Hayes and N. Robinson (Editors)
Elsevier Science Publishers B.V. (North-Holland)
© IMIA, 1991

11 EDUCATION ABOUT IT

11.1 Computer Education for Nursing Staff Managers

E S P Pluyter-Wenting SRN and H B J Nieman BAZIS

University Hospital, Leiden, The Netherlands

Abstract

An increasing need has arisen among nursing staff to take an active part in the discussion on the application of computer systems in the field of nursing. This is particularly with a view to improving quality and increasing efficiency of nursing care. Some knowledge of informatics is essential to succeed in this. This paper describes the developments that lead to a post-graduate course for management nursing staff (approximately 100 hours of classes). The objectives of the course, the way in which it was prepared, its setup, duration, organisation and cost are described. The first course was given late in 1984 and was followed up by intensive evaluation. The results of this first course are dealt with and explained.

Introduction

The majority of all nursing in the Netherlands is trained in accordance with the Government regulated "in-service" training law dating from 1921. Over the years, training has obviously been adapted to our changed society and views, but the basic principle has remained unaltered: practical nursing training in a hospital or institute, backed up by theoretical lessons. In other words a student-nurse carried out nursing duties and receives in return training and a salary. Training takes three and a half years and comprises at least 1,060 hours of lessons and 77 weeks of practical nursing. Since 1972 nursing training is also given on a daytime basis (colleges of higher education). Within the context of this paper it is relevant to mention that Information Science is not taught in any of these courses.

However, since the start of the 1970s informatics has undergone rapid and fascinating development, also in the health care sector. In various areas of nursing the computer has become a valuable asset and it would appear that this trend will indeed continue at a fast pace. Learning to handle and make use of the computer is at least for many young people more or less child's play. Recently basic informatics courses have been included in primary and secondary school curricula, meaning that in some years almost everyone will be acquainted with the working of computers and have at least a basic knowledge of how to use them.

This cannot be said of the generation forming today's working society. This is of course also true of nursing staff; they had already completed their training before the previously sketched developments occurred. And yet it is particularly this generation which is confronted with the question as to whether and how computer technology can be applied in their area of work. The high costs of health care in general force those persons on the management side to give thought to increasing efficiency without allowing a subsequent reduction in quality of work.

Experience elsewhere has taught that computer technology can assist well in this area (O'Connor, 1983).

Making correct use of this technology is in turn also based on expertise, an expertise which at present is lacking on the part of nursing staff managers. It was in fact particularly this aspect that directly lead to the setting up of the first national "Post-graduate Informatics Course for Nursing Staff Management".

This training course serves to provide the student with a knowledge of the possibilities as regards the computer in general, and in particular with regard to its application in the field of nursing. It is intended to provide them with knowledge and insight of the supporting function a computer system can provide in further development and progress in the nursing profession.

In the first instance the course was set up for nursing staff managers considering their leading key-role. To ensure that decisions are taken correctly (also as regards computerisation) nursing staff in supervisory positions must also be trained in this field. They must also be able to participate in the discussions and will be expected to be able to indicate those areas of nursing in which computerisation can offer support and increase quality. They must also be able to evaluate the results of computer applications.

Although extensive discussions were held regarding the possibility of allowing access to the course to the management staff of other health sector disciplines (doctors, physiotherapists, dieticians, etc) it was decided that the course should primarily be open to nursing staff with the objective that particularly this group would feel a sense of involvement. However, there is no objection to others than nurses taking part in the course as long as their number remains limited.

Development

The whole process of development can be divided into a number of different elements.

Initiative and Target Group

The initiative was taken in September 1983 by Chief Nursing Officer, Mrs J J von Nordheim, of the Dutch Ministry of Welfare, Health and Cultural Affairs. At Mrs von Nordheim's suggestion a Curriculum Committee was formed comprising:

  3 computer scientists all working in different areas of health care

  2 nursing officers

1 representative of the Ministry of Health (Chief Nursing Officer)

1 representative of the Ministry of Education and Science

1 external consultant

This committee set itself the objective of setting up and starting a training course in informatics for nursing staff managers within a period of one year. The whole training programme was designed and compiled by the Curriculum Committee and entailed 13 meetings held over a period of 10 months.

Objective
The development of knowledge and insight in the field of:

the basic terminology used in Informatics: the working of, and history of the computer

The analysis of problems and problem solving

future developments and possibilities

the significance of Informatics for:

- nursing practice

- the decision taking process as regards nursing staff management

the social and ethical consequences of computerisation

The central theme of the training course was not to be the actual operation of the computer, but the provision of knowledge into the possibilities and consequences of automatic information processing.

Duration, Content and Structure
After studying literature on this subject, the decision was taken to base the course more or less on the second level of education ("level II") as defined and explained by Ronald (1983). The choice was made for approximately 100 hours of lessons, the argument being that particularly supervisory nursing staff need a more extensive training than the general user to be able to take justifiable policy decisions. Also they will be expected to help towards the development or acquisition of computer systems.

Theoretical Structure
The course was divided into three separate parts:

1 Introduction and hands-on experience (approx. 30 hours)
- - Basic Informatics terminology and the various components of a computer system
- - Becoming acquainted with programming (analytical thinking and the application of algorithms in the form of practical lessons: approximately 11 hours)
- Data storage and representation; the utilisation of data and communication

- Aim and set-up of a hospital integrated information system.

2 Theory and practice of applications in the health care sector in the field of nursing care, management, training and research (approximately 40 hours)
   - survey of present and future applications
      - explanation and demonstration of systems for:

   outpatient appointments

   patient registrations

   drugs distribution

   admission, transfer and discharge

   nursing care plans

   word processing

   computer assisted instruction

   diagnostic related groups

   allocation of student nurses

   patient care classification

   personnel information

   surgical history

   online retrieval of data on patients and nursing procedures

   meal ordering and distribution

3 Various aspects of automation (approximately 30 hours)

   management of automation project

   choice of hardware and software

   cost-benefit analysis

   social and ethical aspects

   data protection and privacy

   participation of nurses in the further development of automation

   technological developments and future possibilities

Teaching Methods, Equipment and Evaluation
Transfer of knowledge via lectures and demonstrations has been chosen as the form of teaching. This method was chosen because of the number of persons taking part (50) and the necessity to convey a large amount of know-how. The course included four practical lessons. The group was divided into two sections during the practical lessons which were aimed at giving the student an idea of the analytical and problem-solving approach adopted when developing software. This was demonstrated to the students by having them develop a simple computer program themselves. These lessons also served to acquaint the students with the actual working of a computer. One microcomputer was available per two students.

During the final practical lesson the students were expected to be able to write a simple program in BASIC to solve a nursing management related problem.

Other teaching methods were impossible to realise apart from a few discussion group sessions due to the group's size. (This was found to be a negative aspect later on.) Special teaching equipment that deserves mention is:

> display terminals (13) for the practical lessons

> a large size video display unit that made it possible via a modem and terminal to facilitate an on-line connection with a hospital computer so that programs could be demonstrated direct. This facility was used in the second half of the training course and proved both illustrative and enlightening.

> a syllabus was also provided during the course which included the various teachers' contributions.

The Curriculum Committee felt the need for learning to be evaluated by a multiple choice examination. It considered allowing the students to write a paper on informatics instead of a multiple choice examination, but this was decided against due to the fact that as well as following the course the students also had a full time job to carry out and an essay could have placed an unreasonable burden on them.

Organisational Aspects

Organisation

With a view to the normal work of the participants it was decided to run the course on a part-time basis. In practice this meant once a week (Monday) over a period of four months. It was also decided that the course should be given in an established training centre as centrally as possible. Six hourly lessons were planned per day and the practical lessons were held in one of the Leiden University Medical Faculty's lecture halls, especially equipped for this purpose.

In order to place the training course within an organisational framework the "Stichting Informatica Opleidingen voor Verpleegkundigen" (S.I.O.V.) [Foundation for Informatics Training for Nursing Staff] was established. The Board of this foundation comprises nine people and carried final responsibility for the whole of the training course. The Board delegated the actual content of the training course to the Curriculum Committee. Direct management and implementation of the course was put in the hands of an organisation advisory bureau. The Board and Curriculum Committee are given secretary support by the University Hospital of Leiden.

Costs

At the Board's request, the Ministry of Welfare, Health and Cultural Affairs awarded a one-time grant of US$3,000 to assist with the initial costs (advertisements, printed matter, legal costs, etc). For the rest, the training course has been financed from study fees at US$800 per person, covering the costs.

Recruitment/Enrolment

Teachers: The Curriculum Committee made the choice of persons to be invited to join the teaching staff. Due to the large number of different subjects to be taught and the specific expertise needed on the part of the teachers, there were a large number of teachers (approximately 50 persons). Each teacher was requested to formulate his or her specific subject matter in writing to facilitate the actual composition of the syllabus. Practically all the teachers were involved with health care automation in one form or another.

Students: Advertisements and notices about the training course were placed in the professional journal for the nurses. Brochures were also printed and distributed on a large scale. Letters went out to all Dutch hospitals. The number of candidates outnumbered the places available and a waiting list had to be drawn up.

Procedure

Participation

The course started on September 3 1984 with 50 participants. A breakdown into groups of different functions, age group and field of work was compiled and is shown below:

a. Function:

8	Director of nursing
18	Division officer
1	Educational officer
5	Assistant Director of Nursing
11	Head Nurse
1	Staff Nurse

b. Age Group:

Average Age 39 years

Age Range 29-58 years

c. Field of Work:

3	Community health care
24	General hospitals
21	University hospitals
2	Nursing homes

From these facts and figures we may conclude that the target group of hospital management staff/nursing staff managers did indeed take part in the course.

Relevant Information
The whole training course went as planned. No one withdrew from the course and the average attendance percentage was above 90%. On each day of the course, the students were requested to complete an evaluation form containing the following questions:
the relevance of the subject to the course as a whole

> content of the lecture

> teacher/lecturer presentation

The student had the choice of awarding scores in the following categories: good/average/poor. These forms were then used for the leader of the course to compile an average score per subject.

A certain amount of unrest was noted among the students halfway through the course as regards the final examination and during a discussion it became clear that the multiple choice exam was regarded with awe by some students. It appeared that would prefer to have the choice of either writing a paper or taking a multiple choice examination. This was sanctioned by the Curriculum Committee.

Results

Final Examination
Since this was the initial start of a completely new training course a great deal of attention was devoted to its evaluation. In addition to the daily evaluation forms referred to earlier, the final evaluation consisted of two separate parts: a written evaluation based on open-ended questions, and an oral evaluation in the presence of members of the Curriculum Committee and the Board.
In the written evaluation the students were asked their opinion on:

> the set-up of the course

> its organisation

> significance of the training as regards one's own work

> teaching method

> any subject not covered, etc

> the need for practical lessons

> method of testing students' knowledge at end of training

> distribution of hours over the different subjects

During the oral evaluation interviews any suggestions that had been put forward were discussed in depth and the strong and weak points of the course were also discussed. Both written and oral evaluation can be summarised as follows:

Strong Points

    the course is well set out and should be continued

    for the greater part the course met expectations

    the set-up of the course, subjects, duration and frequency of lessons have all been given a positive assessment

    the practical lessons were judged to be of great value

    the organisation of the course received positive assessment

    the quality of the syllabus was found to be good

    the course apparently fits in well with the needs arising in the work situation

    the course provided an excellent survey of state-of-the-art automation in the Dutch Health Care Sector

    no subjects were thought to be lacking

Weak Points

    method of teaching was rather one-sided, i.e. lectures were often used; the student remained passive

    due to the large number of different teachers, various parts of lectures tended to overlap

    there was too little opportunity to exchange ideas on experience gained as regards automation in one's own work situation

    there was insufficient time available for some specific nursing subjects

A general need was expressed for a short follow-up course to keep in touch with further developments in this field. There was also the wish expressed that certain specific subjects should be dealt with in more depth, particularly new developments in the nursing profession and possible computer support. Although the approach taken made it possible for us to pass on a great deal of knowledge in compact form, the actual teaching effect was not judged to be optimum.

Final Examination Results

As pointed out earlier, the students were given the choice of either writing a paper or sitting a multiple choice examination. Of the 50 students, 37 took the examination and the others preferred to write a paper.

Some students expressed a wish to write both a paper and sit the examination. Of the 37 candidates, 36 students were awarded sufficient marks for the multiple choice exam. At the time of writing, the results of the papers are not yet known. From the multiple choice examination we are able to conclude that the students have learned a great deal in a short period of time. This is a most significant observation when we consider the number of students that participated in the course.

Conclusion
It has indeed appeared possible to organise a post-graduate informatics course for nursing staff managers in a relatively short period of time. The target group made full use of the opportunity as can be seen from the functions held by the students.
On the whole it would seem that the training course has come up to expectations and deserves to be continued. The next course will be adjusted on a number of points based on recommendations from the students.

References

1. O'Connor, Fotine D 1983, Nurse Management Systems and Budget Control (Medinfo '83, Amsterdam)

2. Ronald, J S 1983, Learning about Computers (Medinfo '83, Amsterdam)

International Primary Care Computing
G.M. Hayes and N. Robinson (Editors)
Elsevier Science Publishers B.V. (North-Holland)
© IMIA, 1991

11.2 Education and Information Technology

Chairman :Prof. Khaihara, University Hospital Computer Center, Tokyo, Japan

Presenter :Mrs E. Pluyter-Wenting, Bazis Foundation PO Box 901 2300 AX Leiden
The Netherlands

Discussant:Mr Alan McWilliams, Dept. of General Practice New Medical School
Ashton Street Liverpool UK

Rapporteur:Chairman's Opening Remarks

The role of information technology in education must be carefully implemented. It is important to consider the duality of the use of computers in education with the education of the computer user. These two fundamental considerations are very much inter dependent. There are four broad categories of people that we have to educate:

- a) Medical students
- b) Medical doctors. In particular, those who qualify before the use of IT becomes incorporated into the medical curriculum. It is hoped that the next generation of doctors will be introduced and become adept at using IT whilst undergraduates.
- c) Allied health personnel
- d) Patients.

Other important items to consider when introducing IT into health care are:

The environment in which computers are sited, i.e. the hospital and at the primary health care level.

The topics to be taught

The ways to teach

The assessment of the effectiveness of the teaching

First Speaker

Discussion from the presentation

The participants at the workshop all agreed that this was a very successful training program, that it met the needs of the nursing professions and would be appropriate to be introduced into the UK. Unfortunately, the programme is written in Dutch.

It was felt that there was a need for IT training for nurses in the UK and at the present time this wasn't being met.

One of the strengths of the course was that it improved the confidence of the user, whilst also improving the skill of the user. It is important for those involved in education in IT not to confuse confidence with skill. Confidence allied with poor skill leads to errors while skill but poor confidence results in under-utilisation.

It was noted that the needs of professionals will change as IT-knowledgeable people enter the profession. It was therefore suggested that the course should also evolve and perhaps it could be possible to plan for an element of evolution into the course, by allocating 5% of the time to new subjects. As an example of evolution it was suggested that the next generation of students might have an awareness and knowledge of the use of IT, but they would have little knowledge and experience of organisational skills and this would be an appropriate subject to be introduced into future IT courses. It was also noted that there was a need for a lower level course.

The workshop commented that it should be remembered that implementation of IT is a continual process and that the computer industry is continually striving to attain higher and faster standards and it is envisaged that IT users will similarly have to incorporate these improvements into the way they work. An element of despair was introduced when it was noted that the UK medical schools are still very slow in introducing and incorporating an IT syllabus into the core curriculum.

One member of the workshop had been involved in discussions with the GMC over the past five years and had noted that some progress had been made in that the GMC are now willing to discuss the idea of IT as being possibly relevant to the undergraduates' needs, but are still a long way from agreeing to its incorporation into a curriculum.

The final point made was that we all must remember that it is not knowledge itself that is important, but the ability to manipulate knowledge usefully.

Second Speaker

The essence of this talk was an amplification of the Chairman's opening remarks. Mrs Osborne gave an insightful overview of the key elements that need to be considered when planning training in IT. From the outset it is important to explain what IT can do, and just as important to explain what it can't do.

How to Educate

We then discussed ways of educating. There should always be an eye on future needs. It is important to understand and thereby differentiate between present needs (and thereby teaching methods) and future needs and methods. To educate, a team approach is best. It should be recognised that the introduction of IT into the primary health care setting can be seen as a tremendous threat by many of the personnel in this field. Therefore a non threatening approach to training will be more suitable. The implementation of an IT training course needs to be rigorous in its planning, especially with respect to its duration and the methods of training to be used. It should be stressed that there is not one correct way of training but one should adopt a "horses for courses" approach.

All the documentation for the course should be well planned and printed and distributed in advance of the start. If possible, try to personalise it. It has been found that students benefit more if an element of feedback and gain is introduced into the design of the course.

When planing, it is important to learn from previous mistakes; not only one's own, but also from those of others who have run similar courses. Feedback from students on the course is an invaluable source of planning information.

There are three major issues in IT education:

> The accumulation of knowledge. This is probably learned best in groups, i.e. lectures.

> The acquisition of skills. This is a much more personal experience and should be taught at a much more individual level.

> The development of attitudes. This is a group or sharing experience, where interpersonal relations are very important.

A particularly valid point that was made was that those doing the training must be adequately trained themselves. It is very common to take "experts" in one field and bestow on them expertises of another field without any foundation. As an example, to be an effective teacher the IT expert must also be trained in communication assessment and other skilis as deemed necessary to teach capably.

There was a short discussion following this presentation which focussed on the lack of infrastructure available for establishing training courses throughout the country for health service personnel, especially in the primary health field. There are approximately thirty thousand GPs in the UK, and each should be employing two full time equivalent ancillary staff. Thus there is a minimum of sixty thousand personnel who will need to be trained in matters of IT, and there is a huge absence of courses or planned courses for them to attend. The PHCSG has collaborated with a commercial company to set up modular courses around the country. This scheme is still in its infancy and has not been fully evaluated. It was felt strongly that there is a large demand for structured learning programmes for GP staff.

The workshop was successful in that it identified the need for effective education in IT within the health care sector. The fundamentals for successfully establishing schemes were discussed and a very successful model from Holland was demonstrated. Have we the influence and tenacity to establish similar schemes in our own countries?

International Primary Care Computing
G.M. Hayes and N. Robinson (Editors)
Elsevier Science Publishers B.V. (North-Holland)
© IMIA, 1991

11.3 Objectives for Education in Medical Informatics

Alan McWilliams,

Lecturer in Clinical Information Science, GP Dept, Liverpool University, PO Box 147
Liverpool, L69 3BX, Phone: 051-794-5602

Introduction

When so much of the healthcare structure is so evidently in need of IT, and hence in need
of education and training in the use of IT, there could be some temptation to address
immediately those areas most prominently visible. There are dangers in this approach,
though; it may lead to poorly focussed effort and wasteful duplication, and will certainly be
difficult to evaluate in context. If we are to be in a position to audit the education process
itself, we must needs specify and agree some objectives for it.

Such objectives will, inevitably, be to some extent context-specific, and the NHS Review
currently taking place in the UK will certainly have a dominant effect on UK thinking. There
will also, however, be common themes and techniques, and these can and should be shared.

One very special aspect of the healthcare context into which IT is being introduced is its
dramatic polarisation. On one hand there are many healthcare workers who still regard
computers with alarm and hostility on both logistical and philosophical grounds. On the
other hand, there are some so patently infatuated with IT that they believe it to be
automatically desirable and self-evidently helpful. Both extremes are unrealistic, and both
need help before they can make good, integrated, and constructive use of IT. This is one of
the challenges of stating our objectives; What are the minimum extra skills and knowledge
required in order for these people to use IT effectively?

Professor Weizenbaum aptly described an example of introducing a new technology and
attempting to educate for its use [1]. In 1888, when telegraphy first enabled people to send
a message coast-to-coast across the US, it was suggested that each school should now teach
Morse code! Futile though this was, the spirit can be seen mirrored today in those who
include the writing of computer programs in courses for healthcare workers. The vast
majority of healthcare workers will never have any need at all for such knowledge.

Background

In order to design education and training, we need to consider the needs of different sectors
of healthcare, and the technologies available and developing.

Those already registered for tertiary education are easily visible - university undergraduates
(medical, para-medical, nursing, ...) and postgraduates, and college students, are already in
a potent framework which has education and research as major objectives. The problems

of changing the medical curriculum should not be under-estimated, but will perhaps decrease with time. The students are reachable, but what do they need?

Less visible, and less lavishly catered for, are the healthcare workers already in post providing healthcare. They have less time available for education and training, and only some of them will be remotely interested in research. What IT knowledge and skills will enable them to perform better? - An embarrassing question, since answering it involves trying to define roles and seeking insights into what is perceived as "better" in these contexts. Healthcare is notorious for its reluctance to address such issues.

There are thus a whole series of separate levels to address, ranging from full-time courses between three and five years long, down to in-service courses which may last only a few days. Figure 1 suggests a framework within which the issues may be considered. The main sectors represented by practice, research, administration, and education; and IT topics divided into generic and domain-specific.

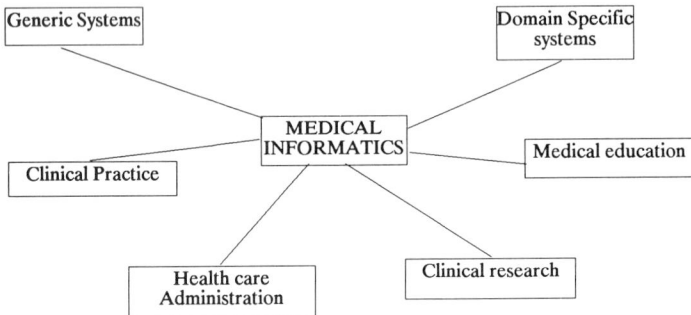

Fig.1. - Medical Informatics in context

Education for Clinical Practice

At each level of healthcare education, at the centre of acute and chronic medical care will be found a strong core of clinical practice. Whatever context supports the education, IT can help in the actual delivery of patient care.

Early examples of such use of IT in clinical practice lie in Intensive Care. Extensive use of automated monitoring and computer processing of results are now a standard feature of the ICU, and it has become virtually impossible to adequately handle patient data as a basis for clinical decisions without direct hands-on use of a computer. Inevitably, this pattern is spreading, and hospitals will have data networks as standard "furniture", with sockets on the wall beside each bed. The clinician needs insight into what information is available to a terminal connected to the network, which subsets are relevant to a current clinical decision, and how to retrieve, process, and interpret the information.

A parallel revolution is taking place in primary health care, where doctors, nurses, and para-medics are beginning to exploit the possibilities of computer-based patient record systems. Many fear the potential effect of introducing a computer into the clinical consultation, and so far medical education does little to reassure. How to retrieve records from a computer, share them with the patient, and use them as a basis for decision-making must become an integral part of training.

Any clinical process will use resources, and generate outcomes in some sense. The enormous variation observable between clinicians and between different clinical processes makes it unlikely that any pre-packaged audit structure will be sensitive enough to be self-sufficient. Each clinician needs to be able to not only store and retrieve information about a clinical process repeatedly undertaken, but to process that information according to rapidly changing and personal criteria. A spreadsheet is the natural vehicle for such individual audit.

As the use of networks to exchange bulk information, and patient-held smart cards to exchange individual records increases it points the need to emphasise our concepts of the medical record as a single logical entity, albeit physically dispersed.

Using a simple network such as videotex just as a retrieval system is a powerful way of overcoming technophobia, since the focus of interest provided by the information rapidly displaces the initial concentration on the technology. OASIS (Online AIDS Support and Information System) [2] has proved a powerful vehicle for conveying a structure of mixed clinical and non-clinical information, and single keystroke operation makes such systems so easy to drive that even the most timid rapidly gain confidence.

Education for Clinical Research

All the components described in (3) above are likewise necessary in an education which will pave the way for clinical research, but can usefully be augmented. Certainly the researcher will put emphasis on the handling of large datasets, and statistical analysis; but increasingly the domain will use graphical techniques, and these must be taught. The humble X-ray is a case in point. As capture, storage, and display of radiographs becomes an essentially digital process, the opportunities for image processing open up. Specifying the processing to be carried out requires insight into what might be possible.

The use of IT also impacts clinical research at its deepest fundamental level. By acquiring the ability to handle large volumes of information, the clinical researcher is enabled to enquire into the very nature of the organisation and processing of clinical knowledge itself. Work on clinical decision-support systems is currently only in its infancy, but will be an important direction for future research.

Education for Healthcare Administration

The fact that healthcare must be administered is inescapable. The persona involved can be argued (the extent of clinician involvement, for example) but the administration process still imposes the need to process data in both individual and aggregate forms.

The ability to use databases to store and retrieve information, and to use tools like spreadsheets to process and represent it, are therefore fundamental. A recent manifestation of this is the advent of geographically-based information systems (GIS) which promise to facilitate resource allocation processing [3,4].

Once strategies have been formulated, they need approval from successive layers in the administration hierarchy. The strategy, the alternatives, and their consequences, must be described and represented, and increasingly this is no longer a task which can simply be passed to somebody else. Computer tools with which to present and communicate information (word-processors, desktop publishers, and presentation packages) are now as indispensable to the administrator as the ability to read and write.

Education - An End in Itself

The obviously visible application of IT to clinical education is that of CAL (Computer Assisted Learning). There are already a considerable variety of CAL packages available commercially - the MAC series [5] of simulation packages, for example. Students at all levels can be encouraged to use computers as both a reference source for course material and also an interactive domain in which they can safely experiment with the likely effects of possible clinical decisions. Whether purchased or self-authored, such packages represent a major commitment of resources, and must be seen to be effective. The graphical capabilities of interactive video are extremely powerful, but demand a correspondingly large investment.

At a simpler level, clinical education itself must be seen as knowledge and information processing. It therefore seems quite natural that we should equip students with the very skills that we would use in our own domain - namely word-processor, database, and spreadsheet. Course notes do not need to be issued on paper, for instance. Issuing them on disc provides prototype notes which can then be edited to the student's taste. Hypertext, and hypermedia in general, are obvious development areas.

Conclusions

In each of the domains visited, the knowledge and skills needed consist of a basic "toolkit" - word-processor, database, and spreadsheet, possibly augmented by insights into domain-specific systems.

In future, it seems likely that secondary (or even primary) education will provide the basic toolkit, but for the moment just providing the toolkit to students and established healthcare workers is a major undertaking. Initially, this should be the focus of endeavour, with insights into domain-specific systems where appropriate. As computer literacy increases the emphasis can be shifted away from the basic toolkit, and greater attention paid to more advanced clinical applications.

References

[1] Weizenbaum, Professor J., speaking at 21st anniversary of National Computing Centre

[2] McWilliams, A, Carey, P. Oasis - Online AIDS Support and Information System. Proc of Current Perspectives in Healthcare Computing - CP88, Brighton, 1988. Roberts, Windsor (eds). Brit. Comp. Soc, with Brit. J. Healthcare Computing; 1988:80-4

[3] Dale, P. GIS. Brit. J. Healthcare Computing, May90;7,4:22-5

[4] Taket, A, Slater, M, Edmonson, D, Curtis, S, Southall, H. The geography of Tower Hamlet's health. Brit. J. Healthcare Computing, May90;7,4:27-9

[5] MAC series of computer simulations: MacPuf, MacPee, MacDope, MacMan. IRL Press, London, 1988

International Primary Care Computing
G.M. Hayes and N. Robinson (Editors)
Elsevier Science Publishers B.V. (North-Holland)
© IMIA, 1991

12   MEDICAL RESEARCH AND IT

12.1   Research Use of Routine Data

Presenter, Dr I E Black

Medical Director, AAH Meditel, Rigby Hall, Rigby Lane, Bromsgrove, Worcs., B60 2EW

Introduction

Very little hard data exist on the very important area of therapeutics relating to the prescribing habits of doctors during the treatment of their pregnant patients. This paper describes an observational, non-interventional study being carried out on all the patients on the AAH Meditel data-base who are recorded as being pregnant during a set period of time. For every patient enrolled there will be a matched control. Analysis will cover the total prescribing information on all patients, with those suffering from asthma, diabetes, epilepsy, hypertension, thyroid disease or liver disease being analysed as a special sub-group. A second study is planned which will go on to follow up the babies born and record, in particular, any occurrence of birth abnormality or the development of a malignant condition.The developing foetus is, or may be, subjected to a wide variety of influences. In particular it is the chemical influences which are the most protean and perhaps the least understood. They may be classified roughly according to the following table.

CLASS	EXAMPLES
Social drugs	Alcohol, marijuana, OCs
OTC drugs	Aspirin, cough remedies
Dietary factors	Food additives
Environmental	
Occupational	Inhaled fumes
Non-occupational	Pollution
Prescription medicines	Anticonvulsants,hypotensives
Endogenous	Hormones

It is in the area of prescription medication that greatest public and indeed professional interest has been centered particularly since the early 1960s when Thalidomide was in use. The term teratogenicity became known to a far wider audience than ever before when some 500 babies were born in the United Kingdom suffering from a characteristic limb deformity which was almost unknown apart from in association with its use during the first few weeks of pregnancy. Of these, approximately 275 survived.In Germany where the drug was incorporated into a wider range of mixtures, including cough remedies, there were approximately 10,000 cases born of whom some 5,000 survived. There followed the formation of The Committee on Safety of Drugs under the Chairmanship of Sir Derek Dunlop which in turn became the Committee on Safety of Medicines. The nature and extent of pre-licence research into medicinal products changed radically with far greater emphasis than before being placed on any possible effects on the foetus of maternal drug intake. The problem however remains that many women who are, or who wish to become, pregnant, are suffering from chronic diseases for which long term therapy is required. What advice does the medical profession have for these women? Should they stop all their medication, should they stop treatment just for part of their pregnancy, is it safe to continue their treatment? Should they be told that they must never risk pregnancy? Clearly there can be no simple answer which will deal with every situation and each case must be decided individually. In some cases it may be vital to maintain the patient's treatment in order to protect the foetus. It is known for instance that babies born to diabetic women who have had good control throughout their pregnancies suffer fewer birth defects than those born to women in whom control was less well maintained.

From where, therefore, is the information available to allow this decision making process to be carried through? Very little data exist. Some prospective studies have been carried on prescribing for pregnant patients. These have been largely confined to long term illnesses such as arthritis, epilepsy or chronic psychiatric disorders. Since they have been performed as intentional studies they have only been able to say what the prescribing patterns of the participating doctors were under study conditions. They have not recorded prescribing patterns on a purely observational and therefore unbiased basis.

Study Design
All patients on the AAH Meditel data-base who are recorded as being pregnant during the study period will be included. The time period has been set so as to accumulate at least twenty thousand pregnancies. Preliminary recruitment figures indicate that the final number available for analysis may be twice this. Patients entered into the study have all their notes and medication retrieved for the period from one year before the pregnancy commenced, throughout the pregnancy and until three months after. For each patient entered, a control will be similarly monitored. Control patients are female patients of the same age who are definitely not pregnant. The control patients will have their notes and medication retrieved over exactly the same period of time as the study patient to whom they have been matched.

Method
The day to day running of the study is achieved by means of a computer algorithm run on the AAH Meditel data-base. This algorithm was tested successfully before the study was commenced.The algorithm looks initially for any code[1] which indicates that a patient is definitely pregnant. Some codes have proved to be ambiguous and have therefore been omitted. For example, last menstrual period (LMP) is used by some doctors to indicate that a patient is pregnant. However, it might also be used when recording data

relevant to a woman who is menopausal. Other codes may be regarded as unambiguous such as the patient's attendance at an ante-natal booking clinic or the recording of a positive result of a pregnancy test. Once the algorithm has identified the patient as being pregnant, it then looks for all other records relating to that patient and in particular looks for any which can assist the accurate dating of the pregnancy such as the result of an ultra-sound scan, or the LMP date. If the patient has already delivered then the date of delivery together with a note of birth maturity of the baby are included in the process.

As has been stated, the patients entered are each matched to a control. These controls are females of the same year of birth who have no note entries indicating any possibility of pregnancy during the study period. All the notes and medication records are retrieved for exactly the same period of time as the study patient with whom they are paired. It is therefore possible that the control will not have been seen by her general practitioner (GP) during the study period and will have no records as a result. Alternative controls were considered. Controls from age matched women who did attend their GP were considered but rejected since this would have biased the control group towards women with some morbidity. Many of the pregnant women entered into the study might not have attended but for the pregnancy.

After full testing and validation of the transmission files and data formats, a short pilot study was successfully run. It is anticipated that analysis of the data will start towards the end of 1990 on this phase of the study. Validation After the study of the computer generated data has been completed, a short validation study will be carried out. This study will select at random a number of practices known to have submitted patient data to the main study. These practices will be visited and all the pregnancies identified from an examination of their records on site. This will allow a check to be made to ensure the transmission to the central data-base of all medication and other important notes. Thus the percentage of pregnancies detected centrally can be validated. In addition it will be possible to check for completeness of the medication record and whether practices have entered hospital data onto the practice computer.

Phase Two
A second study is being planned which will extend on this work with the aim of following up the babies. Since the prescription medication will be known the loop will be closed if the outcome can be measured. In this case the outcome is the baby and a further algorithm will be designed which will look in particular for the incidence of recorded birth defects or malignancy in any of the babies born.

REFERENCES:

Refs., [1] Read Clinical Classification.

International Primary Care Computing
G.M. Hayes and N. Robinson (Editors)
Elsevier Science Publishers B.V. (North-Holland)
© IMIA, 1991

12.2   The Use of a GP Data Bank in Medical Research

Gillian Hall PhD, Mike Allman MBChB

VAMP Research, The Bread Factory, la, Broughton Street, London, SW8 3QJ

The VAMP Research Bank provides a resource of anonymous primary care patient records which can be used for a variety of research purposes. The records are collected from computerised general practices in the United Kingdom where increasing numbers of GPs routinely computerise patient records.

The United Kingdom is an excellent source of data for epidemiology because, within the National Health Service, each person is registered with a general practitioner (GP) who acts as a central agent for the collection and storage of data relating to the health of that person. Until recently, these data were relatively inaccessible because the written records were stored in manual files, and groups of patients could not be readily identified for research purposes. This situation has changed with the introduction of sophisticated computer systems into general practice.

The VAMP Health Computer System

Since 1984, VAMP Health has been a supplier of computer systems to general practitioners. The VAMP Medical system was designed to be used in both the reception area by practice staff and in the consultation room by general practitioners. It is multi-user, allowing data entry and retrieval in every room in the practice. Updated versions of the software are regularly prepared and distributed to VAMP practices.

Four main types of patient information are computerised by practices:

- Basic demographic information, collected when a patient registers, eg age, sex etc.

- Clinical events, including presenting problems, diagnoses and procedures.

- Primary care prescribing with details of drug, form, strength, and dosage.

- Details of preventive medicine.

The information is recorded routinely by GPs, primarily for the purpose of patient care. There is therefore an incentive to record good quality data. As a result of this data recording, each general practice develops its own database of information. VAMP is able to remove this information in an anonymous form and pool it centrally to form the Research Bank.

The VAMP Medical Research Group

In May 1987, the VAMP Medical Research Group was formed. To become part of the Medical Research Group, a practice first buys a VAMP computer system. The doctors in the practice can then sign a second agreement to record patient notes on computer following a Research Protocol. These patient notes are regularly released to VAMP, in an anonymous form. Monthly payments are made to the practice, provided that the data recorded are maintained at the standard required, following an initial 12 month training and familiarisation period. The formation of the Medical Research group has had three major effects.

1. To increase the number of practices in which patient records are computerised.
2. To increase the quality and standardisation of data collected.
3. To formalise the arrangement between VAMP and the GPs, whereby anonymised patient data are copied to VAMP regularly.

The GPs in the Medical Research Group have agreed to collect patient data as defined in a specific Research protocol. On-site training is given to ensure that they fully understand the requirements and a twelve month training and familiarisation period is allowed. Practices are required to record, on all permanently registered patients, demographic details, every therapy prescribed and significant medical problems, including primary and secondary care details.

Collection of Research Data

Every two months, anonymised patient information is collected from the practices. To maintain patient confidentiality, details such as names and addresses are replaced with identification numbers during collection. A patient's date of birth is also removed, but age is recorded by holding year of birth for patients over 5 years old, and month of birth for under 5s. The patient can not be identified by anyone outside the practice. However, it is possible for researchers at VAMP to identify the practice and request that the GP provides more anonymous information for the purposes of validation or follow-up.

Validation

Three levels of validation are routinely conducted on all research information. At the practice level, information from every collection is loaded into a database and a range of analyses conducted. The analyses are designed to monitor two areas; firstly, that the data have been collected properly and, secondly, that the computerisation of patient records follows the Research Protocol. Only data from those practices which pass the validation are entered into the Research Bank.

The second level of validation occurs when the incidence of disease in the Research Bank as a whole is compared with other statistics.

A third level of validation is possible when specific studies are conducted using the Research Bank. Often, during an investigation, it is necessary to refer back to the practice about an individual patient of interest; for example to confirm that a diagnosis was made in hospital or to obtain other details.

By January 1990 there were 1370 practices using VAMP computer systems and 100 systems installed per month. 900 of these, with about 5 million registered patients, are in the Medical Research Group. The majority is currently working through the twelve month maturity time, but in summer, 1989, a Research Bank of over 800,000 patients was available. This is growing rapidly and it is projected that the full 5 million patients will be involved in the scheme by the end of 1990.

Uses of the VAMP Research Bank

The Research Bank is a multi-purpose data resource. Since patient records are computerised routinely and pooled centrally, it is possible to conduct a number and variety of studies at any time. Current uses include:

> Post-marketing surveillance (PMS),
>
> market research,
>
> health service planning
>
> other epidemiology.

PMS is one of the key areas of interest. The Research Bank provides a resource for conducting PMS on new chemical entities, as well as the investigation of drug safety issues relating to established products. PMS functions can be divided into two; hypothesis generation and hypothesis testing.

Observational follow-up studies to generate hypotheses about possible side effects of medicines can be conducted on established products, but are more commonly used to investigate drugs which are newly marketed in the United Kingdom or other countries. The methodology involves identification from the Research Bank of a cohort of patients who have received a prescription for the drug of interest. Clinical events which occur after exposure are examined, and their frequency compared to that in matched reference groups. When required, it is possible to review individual patient records without identifying the patient.

In the second type of study, an hypothesis of an association between a medicine and an adverse event can be tested. The aim of the study may be to calculate the incidence of a problem, to provide information for a product application, to identify whether inappropriate prescribing has caused the problem, or to investigate whether or not a product should be withdrawn from the market. The 3 study design will depend on the hypothesis under investigation and can be by case-control or use the cohort approach. Congenital anomalies can also be studied because mothers and their offspring can be linked.

Use of the VAMP Research Bank for PMS has a number of advantages:

- all general practice medicines can be monitored there is no interference with prescribing because GPs are unaware of which drugs are under investigation.

- the study design is flexible

- fast identification and follow-up of patients is possible - comparator groups can be identified

- patients can be followed up over several years if necessary

- interim analysis of records is possible.

Health Service Planning

The resources of the VAMP Research Bank can also be used for the benefit of the Health Service as a whole. Increasingly, there is a need for high quality data that can be used to provide the clinicians and managers with the information they need to work effectively.

Until now, there has been no regular, reliable source of information on morbidity in general practice, linked to prescribing and health care activity. What information has been available is incomplete or out of date. Even with PACT data, it is not possible to analyse by age and sex.

The protocols for recording information, and the rigorous validation of the data collected, allow confidence in the results of the comparisons that emerge. Haphazard data collection simply results in meaningless data.

The Research Bank can be interrogated to provide analysis by:

> geography eg local area, region or UK
>
> age and sex
>
> disease group
>
> prescribing patterns
>
> use of secondary care facilities trends over time

The uses of the information are many. Examples include:

> identifying health care needs
>
> planning services to meet needs
>
> monitoring the effect of services
>
> planning appropriate preventive services
>
> identifying "at-risk" groups to target services

Conclusions

Primary care computing is more advanced in the United Kingdom than in any other country. The increasing number of computerised general practices in conjunction with the structured National Health Service has facilitated the creation of the VAMP Research Bank, an innovative research resource which can help answer a number and variety of questions. These questions are of relevance to the pharmaceutical industry, the National Health Service, regulatory authorities and academia.

International Primary Care Computing
G.M. Hayes and N. Robinson (Editors)
Elsevier Science Publishers B.V. (North-Holland)
© IMIA, 1991

12.3 THE EXETER CARE CARD PROJECT

Dr Robin J Hopkins

The Department of General Practice, University of Exeter, Postgraduate Medical
School, Barrack Road ,Exeter, EX2 5DW

The Exeter Care Card Project is a Department of Health sponsored pilot trial to investigate
the potential for a patient retained medical smart card record within the National Health
Service.

It has long been recognised that the essence of good patient care is provided by good record
keeping. Shared care within the Health Service requires shared information handling and
for NHS planning to be effective the information needs to be retrievable and contain
common data sets. [1]

At the British Computer Society Meeting in Oxford in the Autumn of 1988 John Shaw, the
chairman of the Family Practitioner Services Computer Strategy Steering Committee,
outlined the Department of Health Strategy for networking within the NHS. This involves
the production of a continuous integrated network to link all Family Practitioner Service
Regions, the central NHS register, the Prescription Pricing Authority and the Dental
Estimates Board with all GPs, Opticians and Dentists.

The current Health Service review and its associated white paper "Working For Patients"
recognises the need for an efficient information sharing system in order to improve
efficiency and help contain costs and declarations are made regarding the provision of funds
to implement such new systems.

There are many problems associated with networking not the least of which is the
introduction of protocols to allow the many and varied systems to communicate. Of
necessity any computer system used within the Health Service environment should be
capable of providing immediate access to information about the Patient and facilitate the
interchange between the health care professional and Patient whilst at the same time
maintaining confidentiality of this information. Large databases at different sites accessed
by a networking system could meet this requirement, although they necessitate significant
financial commitment. However, one of the fundamental issues is the communication of
confidential information about individual patients over what is essentially an open access
network. Ethically it is reasonable to allow depersonalised information collated from
groups of patients, ie planning data, to be communicated over such a network but it is of
more concern with regard to individual patient data. [2]

Inevitably within a service as diverse as the N.H.S. there will be sites that are not served by
the N.H.S. network and a complimentary system is necessary that allows communication of
individual patient data, without making it available to all network users and preferably
making it patient controlled. The necessity for such a system means the patient has to be

able to carry around with him portable computerised media which can communicate with any other system.

Any computer system used within the Health Service environment should be capable of providing immediate access to information about the patient and facilitate the interchange between the health care professional and patient whilst at the same time maintaining confidentiality of this information. With its inherent security and portability, the Smart Card is able to provide confidentiality of information exchange, and still provide the necessary linkage required to set up a comprehensive data management system.

Exeter University Postgraduate Medical School's Department of General Practice was approached by the Department of Health in the Autumn of 1987 to examine the feasibility of using a Smart Card medical record within the Health Service. Smart Card medical records have been in use in Europe for some time, despite few European general practices having computers and a trial of Patient portable computerised media was undertaken in Pontypridd in 1986 [3]

System Design

Despite the excellent work previously carried out, none of the systems already developed matched the potential needs of the National Health Service, as previously outlined. A large number of computer systems are already in existence within the Health Service and a proliferation of general practice, pharmacy and dental systems already exist, all operating with different languages and operating systems. It was therefore necessary to devise a communicating medium which acts as an interpreter between all these individual data bases and allows the passage of information from one data base to another. This, of necessity, means that the portable computerized record is a sub-set of clinical inform@ion stored at varying sites within the Health Service and has to carry information independently from the host data base over an unpredictably routed network. [4]

A working partnership was created by the Department of Health, involving the Department of Health, Exeter University, Bull and Abies Informatics with the added support of AAH Meditel and Datacard UK with the intention of designing and building such a communicating network to investigate the potential use of a Smart Card record within the Health Service. The Care Card system user specification and resulting design was drawn up by the Department of General Practice, Exeter University over the months at the end of 1987 and set out to produce a computer system with sufficient flexibility for the Health Service.

The design requirements were:

      1. that the system should be totally secure.

      2. allow graded levels of access to information appropriate to the user.

      3. patients could be allowed to view data contained within their own card.

4. that it should be possible to transmit clinical information, laboratory information, patient details, and prescribing information via this medium and that there should be no limitations as to the type of clinical information carried on the card.

It became necessary to define a global record structure that enabled subsets of information to be extracted as required. Such a global structure was termed "the effective data set" and is made up of a theoretically infinite number of basic data sets. Such a record structure had to be capable of storing data in all these areas using a unified coding system. The Exeter Care Card's effective data set is outlined below and caters for all health care needs identified so far, with the exception of the transmission of financial information.

Effective Data Set:

Registration details

Ethnic group

Religion

Language spoken

Health Care Professional Identifiers

Medication / Prescribing Details

Allergies / Sensitivities

Symptoms

Examination findings

Diagnostic findings

Laboratory data

Employment details

Administration data

Emergency data (including donor Status)

The use of such a comprehensive data set necessitates the use of an equally comprehensive coding structure. Evaluation of the currently available coding systems revealed only one solution to such a requirement - that of the use of the Read Clinical Classification.

In order to allow the unambiguous communication of data within such a network and to enable data to be used for Health Service planning a common data coding system has to be used. The Care Card is designed to store data using the five character alpha-numeric Read Clinical Classification.[6] The use of such a classification means that computer routines can be written which make use of its hierarchical nature.

Specific algorithms can be written to address the processor on the card, which is then able to present only data specifically required for the production of the computerised shared care format, as well as the full data set on request.[7]

As well as the use of the Read classification, a data compression technique devised by Bull is utilised in order to maximise the potential of the Care Card for storage of medical information.

Software

For the purposes of the Care Card Trial a common set of clinical information Software is provided by ABIES Informatics who have worked in conjunction with Bull on implementation of the Software design. During the course of the trial it has become apparent that at the pharmacy sites in particular, the original user specification and its resultant system did not allow for sufficient flexibility of use. As a result of this a new bespoke pharmacy system has been written by The Clinical Information Consultancy and introduced at these sites. All the above systems are equipped with a comprehensive drug interaction system, plus a pharmaceutical lexicon.

System Security

In built security within the Smart Card plus the ability to transfer data from its chip to the host system based software routines provides the ultimate security application - Health Care professionals are issued with key cards that enable terminals and allows them to have access to the Care Card accessing system. Information about the user is passed from the key card to the host system software that allows graded access to the host system and the data contained on the card. Existing hardware security and software passwords are maintained. Each key card is p.i.n. Protected, as is the patient's own Care Card, the key card effectively bypassing the need for a Patient's p.i.n. with respect to accessing data contained on the Care Card.

Levels of Access

Access to data contained on the Care Card is determined by codes built into the key card and functionality of the overall system is determined by an interplay of Security statements contained on the key card and by software routines built into the host system and Care Card. The system is designed in such a manner that doctors have total access to all the data contained on the card. Other users have access to data appropriate to their health care needs.

Hardware

The Care Card is a CP8 Smart Card manufactured by Bull France and contains 16k EPROM memory. The chip has its memory effectively divided into three areas:

A secret area - which controls in built security of the card and ensures that any correctly identified protocols are allowed to access data within the other ANO areas of memory. It also contains the coding password section which allows grading of access to data and lastly controls the in-built security system of the card that ensures that the data is permanently locked if the chip is mechanically or electrically interfered with.

An open access area - which identifies the card and certaincharacteristics peculiar to it, i.e. the card number.
A Secure area - Access to this area is "password" protected and graded by software contained within the secret area and within the Care Card contains all the clinical and patient information.

GP sites utilise Hewlett Packard Vectra personal computers provided by AAH MEDITEL and at all other sites Bull machinery is used.

Patient names are imprinted on the card plastic using a new technique provided by Datacard UK which increases legibility.

The Trial

Nine thousand Patients in the Devon town of Exmouth (population thirty-five thousand) have been issued with a Care Card. Patient groups are chosen as follows:

1. All the Patients of a small group practice to enable a study of the use of the communicating system as if the whole Health Service were users)
2. The under fives and the over Sixty-fives of a large group practice the high usage group)
3. Every diabetic in Exmouth

The equipment is available to both read and write to the card at both the above group practices, Exmouth hospital, Exeter main hospital, a large dental practice within Exmouth and every pharmacy in Exmouth. Information was entered on the card at the GP sites at the state of the trial and Patients issued with a card containing a summary record. Thereafter at every encounter with a health care professional, patients have the opportunity to present the card and the data it contains to that professional, who also has the opportunity to add data to it for passage to another health care professional.

The ability for Patients to view the data contained on their own Care Cards is provided at the GP sites participating in the trial. Cards which are lost or become full can be re-issued at the GP site.

At each interplay (card read) of the card data base with the host system data base, the information they contain is compared. Any new or changed data is automatically brought to the attention of the health care professional and updated on the host system database.

Because of the coding system and comparison techniques used, the Care Card is capable of storing in the order of 92 diagnoses plus 27 medicines, all of which can be issued multiple times. Patient name and address can be changed multiples of times.

Evaluation

Evaluation of the trial is being carried out by an evaluation committee, headed by an evaluation manager appointed by the Department of Health and is looking at the system for the one year trial period from the lst March 1989 onwards. The trial is being evaluated with respect to the following:

1. Attitudes of patients and staff.
2. Costs - capital revenue and data loading.
3. Data transmission - accuracy, reliability and speed.
4. Data accuracy - comparison of data provided by Patient verbally and that contained within their care card system.
5. System reliability.
6. Card interaction rates.
7. Health Care effects.

A formal report will be published at the end of the trial which will address all the above areas; however the data analysed and reported here has been obtained from only one of the ANO trial practices and is intended to be an interim report rather than a presentation of the final evaluation.

Demography

In order to evaluate the Care Card, a pilot area was chosen which would allow the fullest possible evaluation to be made of the Care Card system as if the whole Health Service were using this method of communication. Investigation revealed that Exmouth had a closely defined sub-service which referred outside the town only when specialised services or equipment were required. This enabled the trial to be carried out in a contained environment.

Exmouth is the fastest growing town in the South West of England, the population having risen from 8,000 to 34,000 over the last 20 years. The area has a higher than average proportion of the elderly, being a retirement area, with the bulk of the retirees coming from London, Bristol and the Midlands. [8]

Hardware

The computer used for the trial, Hewlett Packard Vectra at GP sites and Bull PCs at other sites, have proved themselves reliable in a testing environment. Card readers (Bull model no TLP 224) have proved equally reliable. Early on in the evaluation it appeared that there was a problem with the type of Smart Card in use. This has not proven to be the case and the cause of failure is interesting to note.

After cards had been personalized and initialized, they were placed in an envelope, along with accompanying letters and mailed directly to the Patient - the card being loose in the envelope. After ANO months of the trial it became apparent that the card failure rate was greater than the design specifications and far higher than that experienced in European projects to date. Direct observation and electrical analysis of the chips revealed that faults were related to trauma.

As a result of this Bull carried out an analysis of the British postal system involving direct observation of automated sorting, franking and postcoding machinery and a trial post and testing of cards, with the card being placed in different relative positions in the envelope. Examination of the automatic post coding machines revealed that envelopes were being subjected to acute bending stress (potentially outside ISO standards) and that this was a possible cause of failure. Analysis of cards held in envelopes in different relative positions revealed that cards held in the middle of the envelope longitudinally were subjected to less stress and were less liable to damage by the postal system. As a result of this Data Card UK have been able to design and supply paper card carriers for transportation of Care Cards whilst in standard envelopes.

Costs

One of the major fears about doctors implementing computer systems in general practice has been the hidden costs of data management. The following figures are obtained over a ten year period of recording at this site.
Average time taken to summarise LLoyd George envelope (Sample size 4,000) using receptionist and nurses to produce summaries:

    - 17 minutes per record

Average time taken to load computer summary onto ABIES/AAH Meditel system per record (Sample size 4,000):

    - 8.6 minutes

Average time taken to maintain database, enter hospital letters, lab reports etc, per thousand patients per day:

    - 15.6 minutes

Average time taken to issue a Care Card from prepared data base (sample size 4,009):

    - 2 minutes

A manpower effect at the doctor's site described in this paper has been the time saved in reduced filing time - the paper record not being utilized at this surgery. Staff response has been more than favourable over the whole range of staff (ages 22 - 70) and no difficulty has been found in using the system by those personnel who had not previously used a computer.

Consultation Effects

Another fear is that of the computer interfering in the doctor patient relationship and slowing down the consultation.

Analysis of consultation length with both partners using the computer have produced the result that whilst the use of a computer on its own prolongs the consultation slightly initially there is no statistically significant difference between consultation lengths before the introduction of a desk top computer and its use during the consultation, with the addition of a Care Card.

Health Care Effects

Analysis has been made of work patterns and the performance indicators as described by Higginson [9] have been used throughout the trial period.

The practice showed no drop in overall consultation rates. However the number of new visits requested of the practice fell from 90 to 75 per month, as did the number of telephone consultations, dropping from 86 to 56 per month.

The number of patients referred from the practice to hospital during the period was not significantly altered. However there was a marked reduction in the number of investigations being carried out, particularly in chemical pathology and haematology. Pre care card 7% of consultations would result in an investigation being carried out. Post care card the level has fallen to 7.2% (aggregated data). With reference to prescribing costs the number of repeat prescriptions per month per 1,000 Patients, the number of items on them and their cost have fallen:

Pre care card 98 scripts/1,000 patients/4 week period

     9 items per script

Post care card 132 scripts/1OOO patients/4 week period

     8 items per script

Average cost per item fell by 1% on repeat prescriptions.

This has been assessed over a period when the FPC average has risen by 3% with no change in the practice formulary

At the time of writing there is still a large amount of data to be analysed for the second GP practice and other Health Care Professionals.

Summary

The trial has produced a large amount of information about data management over the Health Service area covered by Exeter. We have learnt a great deal about the way the Health Service actually works and gained valuable insight into the potential information needs of the service. The technology appears to have proved itself in a testing environment and the potential for a "soft network" provided by a smart card seems to have been demonstrated.

References

1. Korner Committee Reports H.M.S.O.

2. Goble C. and Kay S. Protection and Control of information in Medical Databases. Pulling Together - Current Perspectives in Health Care Computing 1988.

3. Stevens R and Crabbe A. "Credit card" medication records: The Pharmaceutical journal. December 1988

4. Markwell.D. Software integration of smart cards with an existing clinical information system. Proceedings of Smart Card 89.

5. Information Handling in General Practice 1988. ed.Westcott and Jones ISBN 0-7099-5228-7

6. Read J. and Benson T. Comprehensive Coding: British Journal of Health Care Computing. Volume 3. No 2. May 1986. Pg 22-25

7. Hopkins R.J. Shared Care a la' Exeter Care Card - Proceedings of Information Technology For Shared Care, British Medical Informatics Society, 10/89.

8. Glyn-Jones A. Growing older in South Devon towns - Univ. of Exeter 1975

9. Higginson B. information for Doctors.- Information handling in General Practice. ed.Westcon & Jones ISBN 0-7099-5228-JG

FINAL PLENARY SESSION

WORKSHOP 1   INTERFACING DOCTORS TO COMPUTER SYSTEMS

MIKE FITTER

It was felt that there was a need for consulting room interface. The system must give something back to the user.   Data transfers within the Health Service and Hospitals have implications for data standards. The implications of using information which had been transferred from one system to another need consideration if there are no standards.

WORKSHOP 2   DECISION SUPPORT

BOB JOHNSON

There are two ways of assessing support validation.   Integration of knowledge based systems. Problem of patients ending up in wrong domain and merging into area of expert system for diagnosis. Question of misconceptions usually as misread diagnosis had been overlooked. Increasing importance of Primary Care. Devolving services to Primary Care area would make a large
economic impact.

WORKSHOP 3 CODING

ANTHONY NOWLAN

The situation is volatile. There are many views and opinions. Clear need for resolving major problems in certain areas. Problems of perceived needs e.g. for creating notes, uncertainty as to how to include these in the notes. Aggregation of large amounts of data when not clear, if agreement with originator of notes.

Nomenclature - classification for aggregation.
Read classification - nomenclature rather than coding may be more appropriate description.
Need to clarify purpose of codes and benefits from them. It was suggested that this be looked at in further sessions.

WORKSHOP 4 SCREENING

BERNARD RICHARDS

1. Opportunistic call for patients - computer provides suitable prompts, even if not very computerised.
2. Check list of what should be done during screening itself.
3. Family history patient completed questionnaire
4. Benefits of screening - this could be linked to smart cards.

WORKSHOP 5 MEDICAL AUDIT

STEPHEN KAY

Five points from Sheldon 1982
1. Set clinical objectives
2. Information collection and analysis
3. Evaluate process and outcome of care
4. Review objectives of clinical care
5. Repeat process to monitor change

Medical practice and audit don't match readily, sociological, political and technical problems. Medical collection of routine data could be the basis from which we could start.

Problems came up to which we should give special attention and the audit process should be cyclic - results repeated, readjusted, fed back and redone.

Audit: "shared care, a searching examination contrasted to the day of Judgement".
"'Lor bless you I can't audit any more than I can audit. I am not accurate". C. S. Lewis.
"Hell is always inaccurate".

WORKSHOP 6 COMMUNICATIONS

PAUL GROB

The European standards are nice as there are so many you can choose between them. Link of hospitals using OSI. OSI standards with the background of the White Paper for further development. Smart cards may lead to a reduction in prescribing. There is no sign of a common technology emerging.
Problems of confidentiality - potential for malignant misuse is enormous (Rupert Fawdry).

Technology much larger to implement than expected.

WORKSHOP 7 THIRD WORLD IT

PROF. ZEF IBRAHIM

"The Third World" constitutes 80% of humanity. Originally all were assumed to be in "one basket", but this is no longer the case, these countries are very different. Regions need to be considered more than countries. China and India are now opening to computer technology.

Literacy and numeracy - only 30% of the world is literate. A quantum jump is possible via IT. Computer technology needs marrying of one technology to another, e.g. with computer and video disc projects opening up.

IT is the engine of change in many regions e.g. Eastern Europe.

Sociological and philosophical aspects are discussed. No general solutions, but the human aspect is more important than technology itself.

Specific needs for particular areas and situations Does power corrupt?

A top downwards approach is preferred by bureaucracies, but a bottom upwards is preferred by the people. Power corrupting, as is control of people who are illiterate.

WORKSHOP 8 DEMOGRAPHY AND IT

GEOFFREY DOVE

Only 1981 census information is available to assess deprivation: Individual resources are only used where deprivation was high. The country was divided into 5000 wards to determine which was a deprived area.

Suggested that GPs decided what were deprived areas. Various deprivation indexes e.g. position of toilet and whether kitchen included in number of rooms determined the allocation of resources.

Suggestion that in two years' time information to FPCs would go to Health Authorities, must be careful not to give too much information as this could be used inappropriately.

WORKSHOP 9 MEDICAL RECORDS

ALAN RECTOR

Alan Rector felt for the first time in such a group that the questions of whether and why we should do it did not need to be raised. There was a consensus that the entire medical record needed to be computerised.

The computerised record was seen as a way of making life easier.

The worry about intrusion was perhaps more one of the Doctor's concerns rather than that of a patient, and maybe the manual riffling through papers was more intrusive to the consultation. The concept of the total record was good if well done, as at the moment what was available was not up to it.

Back-up and reliability were very important. Mustn't trust too much, although more reliable backup may not work and suppliers do not enforce greater security.

Information should be made attributable, as at present most systems do this in only a rudimentary way.

Side effects - much better letters back, as better letters to Consultants are produced. Depends on referral letters and quality of that.

WORKSHOP 10 SECURITY AND DATA PROTECTION

RORY O'MOORE

1. Adopt six safety principles.
2. Need to be tighter on definitions e.g confidentiality and security.
3. Need reference model for health.
4. Develop security/confidentiality audits.
5. Develop security awareness
6. Develop security for education.
7. Define security of access.
8. Define security of transmission - get what paid for.
9. Define risk analysis CCTA risk analysis and methodology.
10. Develop codes of practice for health care professionals.

Final need for new working group to deal with security standards.

WORKSHOP 11 EDUCATION AND IT

IAN GOODMAN

How, what and who should be taught?. Considering how the Dutch programme for teaching Senior Nursing staff - a modular course for 50 nurses per year - lectures, hands on etc - was found to be useful.

Considered wider implications for Doctors, nurses and other health care staff. Considered what can be taught. Doctors and staff need to be taught as well as those that train them, particularly in fields outside their normal ones. A concerted approach is needed.

CONCLUSION:

This letter was prepared at the end of the Working Conference and sent to The IMIA Board.

Primary Health Care Specialist Group of the British
Computer Society,
3 Beech Ave. North, Worcester WR3 8PX, United Kingdom
Fax +44 905 56817

IMIA Working Conference
2-5th April 1990. Brighton, England.

During this weeks conference we have focused on many issues relating to Primary Care Computing and have examined this material in detail in twelve workshops concerned with the following topics:-

1. Interfacing Doctors to Computer Systems.
2. Decision Support
3. Coding
4. Screening
5. Medical Audit
6. Communications
7. IT for Development
8. Demography & IT
9. Medical Records
10. Security & Data Protection
11. Education about and through IT
12. Research Use of Routine Data

This material is being developed into a monograph but meanwhile we would like to record our recommendation that IMIA should reconstitute Working Group 5 as an IMIA Technical Committee under IMIA bye-laws with the following objectives.

Working Group 5 : Primary Health Care Informatics.

Objectives

1. To provide a multi-professional environment for the monitoring and exchange of information about activities in Primary Care Informatics world wide.

2. To foster research and development in Primary Care Informatics, taking into account the regional, political and cultural variances in approaches to primary care.

      3. To foster the development of educational materials and opportunities
          for spreading the awareness of Primary Care Informatics.

4. To assist in the furtherance of the WHO aims of primary care worldwide.

It is suggested that a small steering group is set up to
initiate the establishment of Technical Committee 5 and this
group should consist of S. Kaihara, Rolf Engelbrecht, Glyn
Hayes, Michael Crampton, G.Brauer, with the addition of a
representative from IMIA-LAC. It is further suggested that
the co-ordinator of the group should be Glyn Hayes.

 signed by

        S.Kaihara, Japan. Past President, IMIA

        W.Abbott, Hon.Fellow, IMIA

        B.Barber, UK

        G.Hayes, Chairman IMIA Working Conference,2-5th April 1990,

        R.O'Moore, Ireland

        O.Rienhoff, FRG

Signed on behalf of the above,

S.Kaihara.
Past President,IMIA.

The Future:

The IMIA Board considered the above recommendation. At the meeting of the full IMIA Board held in Glasgow, Scotland in August 1990 the Board agreed to reinstate Working Group 5. In the first instance this would be as a full Working Group until it can consider its functions in details. A further proposal will be submitted to the IMIA board after the Working Group has formalised its activities.

The IMIA Board appointed Dr Glyn Hayes, Chairman of the British Computer Society, Primary Health Care Specialist Group, to be the Chairman of IMIA Working Group 5. His address is:
3 Beech Avenue North, Worcester, England, WR3 8PX. Tel +44 905-54705 Fax +44 905-56817

The first task was to complete these Proceedings. After that the IMIA representatives from each country will be circulated to ask them to propose names of individual workers from their own countries who they consider would be suitable to sit on Working Group 5. Once the names have been collected the Working group can determine the way forward.

In the first instance communications will be by fax and mail. I hope that the first full meeting of the Working Group will take place at MEDINFO 92 to be held in Geneva. Before then I hope that we will have collected a large database of information about the activities taking place in the member countries. This database will be collated in the UK and be available to anyone who wishes to see what is happening around the world in Primary Care Computing.
It will have the following functions.

1. To provide the means of linking workers from different countries who have similar interests.

2. To provide information which individuals can use to apply pressure to governments and other authorities to develop Information technology in their own country.

3. To foster the development of data standards and coding systems to enable international communications of medical information.

Glyn Hayes

12th January 1990

COMPUTERS IN PRIMARY HEALTH CARE

A BIBLIOGRAPHY.

Simon Ashton Towler.

CONTENTS

MEDICAL RECORDS

[2]Abrams ME: Computer terminals in a health centre. Community Health **3**: 81-85, 1971.

[3]Abrams ME: Health Services and the computer. Real time computing in general practice. Health Trends **4**: 18-20, 1972.

[8]Anderson J: Clinical Records System: An Overview. Current Perspectives in HC. 107-114, BJHC, 1984.

[9] Anderson J, Forsythe J: Information Processing of Medical Records. North-Holland, 1970.

[26]Barber JH: Computer assisted recording in general practice. JRCGP **21**: 726 - 736, 1971.

[29]Bassoe CF: A Combinatorial Diagnostic System for General Practice: Evaluation of the Social Impact of Disease by a Computerised Medical Record. MIE 88: 212-214, Springer-Verlag, 1988.

[30]Bassoe C, Sorli W: A Problem-Oriented Computerised Medical Record worked whereas a Chronological did not. MIE 88: 190-199, Springer-Verlag, 1988.

[33]Beilin LJ et al: Computer-Based Hypertension Clinic Records: A Co-operative Study. BMJ **2**: 212,216, 1974.

[35]Billiet R, De Norre L: Comparative research, prevention and audit in general practice using the system oriented registration method. MIE 85: 368-372, Springer-Verlag, 1985.

[36]Billet R: System oriented registration in general practice. MIE 84: 546-551, Springer-Verlag, 1984.

[41]Borst F et al: MEDIAL: a natural language processing system for medical records. MIE 84: 128-133, Springer-Verlag, 1984.

[45]Bradshaw-Smith JH: A computer record-keeping system for general practice. BMJ **1**: 1395-1397, 1976.

[54]Bulpitt CJ et al. Randomised controlled trial of computer-held medical records in hypertensive patients. BMJ **1**: 677-679, 1976.

[58]Cerutti S: The automatic treatment of the information in the medical records at the level of the general practitioner. MIE 82: 303-305, Springer-Verlag, 1982.

[62]Cobbs JS, Miles DP: Estimating list inflation in a practice register. BMJ **287**: 1434-1436, 1983.

[66]Cormack J: The General Practitioners Use of Medical Records. Edinburgh University, 1970.

[68]Crambie DL: Record linkage in automated systems. JRCGP **31**: 325-326, 1981.

[101] Doroba A, Leligdowicz A: Two year experience in problem oriented records of primary health care. MEDINFO 77: 479-480, North-Holland, 1977.

[105] Downs SM et al: Automated Summarisation of On-Line Medical Records. MEDINFO 86: 800-804, North-Holland, 1986.

[108] Dvergsdal P: Interactive patient record. MIE 85: 404-409, Springer-Verlag, 1985.

[110] Ewins DL et al: Computerised updating of clinical summaries: new opportunities for clinical practice and research. BMJ **297**: 1504-1506, 1988.

[111] Farmer RD, Grosc KW: An automated records system for general practice. Br J Prev Soc Med **26** (3): 148 - 152, 1972.

[133] Grant D: Record linkage in general practice: the computers in medical records. Practitioner **204**: 444 - 5, 1970.

[138] Gruer KT: Livingstone New Town - Using a computer for general practice records. JRCGP **22**: 100-107, 1972.

[139] Gruer KT, Heasman MA: Livingstone New Town - Use of computer in general practice medical records. BMJ **2**: 289-291, 1970.

[140] Gunner C: The implications of smart card technology. Current Perspectives in HC: 236-240, BJHC, 1988.

[145] Hannay DR, Mitchell S: Storing Summary Patient Data as a Microcomputer File. JRCGP **35**: 525-526, 1985.

[151] Henderson J: Instant age-sex register. BMJ **288**: 1967-1968, 1984.

[153] Grene JD: Computer Compatible records in general practice. JRCGP **19**: 29-33, 1970.

[155] Heyrman J: Computerisation of the medical record of the general practitioner: systematic registration at each patient-gp contact.MIE 78: 101-108, Springer-Verlag, 1978.

[170] Johnson RA: Computer analysis of the complete medical record including symptoms and treatment. JRCGP **22**: 655-660, 1972.

[175] Kopjar B et al: A micro computer based problem-oriented medical record system for PHC. MIE 88: 207-210, Springer-Verlag, 1988.

[176] Kumpel Z: Referral letters - the enclosure of the general practitioner's computerised record. JRCGP **28**: 163-167, 1978.

[178] Law J: Sell your practice data at profit. Medeconomics: June 1987.

[180] Lawrence M: A computer generated patient carried health check card. JRCGP **36**: 458-460, 1986.

[184] Linnarsson R: Development and evaluation of a complete computer-based problem-oriented medical record system for primary care. MIE 87: 209-214, EDI Press, Rome, 1987.

[185] Lipman EO, Preece JF: A pilot on-line data system for general practitioners. Comput Biomed Res **4** (4): 309 - 406, 1971.

[186] Lloyd SC: Computer-generated progress notes in an automated POMR. J Med. Syst. **8**(1-2): 35-42, 1984.

[192] Malmberg BG: A complete medical record system and its Data Dictionary, used by General Practitioners and district nurses, working in a district health centre. MIE 87: 215-224, EDI Press, Rome, 1987.

[193] Mann N: Smart Cards in Health Care: A solution in search of a problem. MEDINFO 89: 1151-1155, North-Holland, 1989.

[199] McDonald CJ et al: Reminders to physicians from an introspective computer medical record. A two year randomised trial. Ann Intern Med 100(1): 130-138, 1984.

[203] Meldrum D: Simple Computerised Disease Register. BMJ 282: 191-194, 1981.

[224] Preece JF, Hearson JR: The synopsis record card: a stepping stone to the computer. JRCGP 36: 564-566, 1986.

[240] Rawlins D: Development of a family linkage program. Current Perspectives in HC: 31, BJHC, 1989.

[248] Rector AL et al: A survey of developments in medical records and information systems in the UK. MIE 78: 91-100, Springer-Verlag, 1978.

[249] Rector Al, Sheldon MG: Privacy, data decay and the long term medical record. MIE 82: 686-691, Springer-Verlag, 1982.

[250] Reed RC: Transferring documents from one system to another. Comput Nurs 7(2): 58-60, 1989.

[251] Reekie D et al: Handling information in general practice - using feature cards with computers. JRCGP 25: 369-372, 1975.

[252] Reekie D, Horden K et al: New approaches to info handling in general. BMJ 2: 162 - 166, 1974.

[275] Saul PD: Accessing remote data bases using micro computers. JRCGP 35: 384-386, 1985.

[283] Sheldon MG: Giving patients a copy of their computer medical record. JRCGP 32: 80-86, 1982.

[287] Simon P, Naszlady A: Memory Card - Micro Chip - In Primary Health Care. MEDINFO 86: 1015-1018, North-Holland, 1986.

[288] Singer G, Hall G: Results of a Primary Health Care Data Base. Current Perspectives in HC: 48, BJHC, 1989.

[294] Stevens RG, Crabbe AM: Computerised Patient Retained Records: A Working System. Current Perspectives in HC: 250-261, BJHC, 1985.

[296] Stimson DH et al: A problem-oriented information system for a primary care group practice. MEDINFO 77: 463-466, North-Holland, 1977.

[305] Temmerman G et al: PLUSOMR - A microcomputer POMR-SYSTEM for Primary Care. MEDINFO 83: 1173-1176, North-Holland, 1983.

[306] Temmerman G, Plumans W: A modular integrated medical record for general practice. MIE 79: 261-271, Springer-Verlag, 1979.

[318]Van Egmond J, Wieme RJ: COMPADOS: How to convince a physician to use a computerised medical record system. MIE 78: 339-349, Springer-Verlag, 1978.

[319] Vansteenland H: MEDOC: medical documents on computer. MIE 84: 558-564, Springer-Verlag, 1984.

[322] Watkins GB: Computerisation of a diabetic clinic records. BMJ **281**: 1402-1403, 1980.

[332] Anon: The impact of a micro computer on a practice immunisation clinic. The Practitioner **232**: 197, 1988.

[353] Anon: Seizing the opportunity. Practice Computing **3**(1): 23-24, 1984.

[387] Anon: Two-year experience in problem oriented records of primary health care. MEDINFO 77: 479-480, North-Holland, 1977.

[403] Anon: Combined computer generated discharge documents and surgical audit. BMJ **292**: 816-818, 1986.

CONFIDENTIALITY / DATA PROTECTION

[20]Bakker A, Louwese C: Considerations on the Effectiveness of Protection by Passwords. MIE 85: 343-346, Springer-Verlag, 1985.

[24]Barber B: Getting Our DP act together. BJHC **4** (5): 32-36, 1987.

[25]Barber B: Wanted: A Confidentiality Clause in Staff Contracts. BMJ **2**: 702, 1973.

[68]Crambie DL: Record linkage in automated systems. JRCGP **31**: 325-326, 1981.

[96]Dinklo JA: Confidentiality of Medical Data in the Usage of Data Banks. MEDINFO 74: 181-187, Almqvist & Wiksell, 1974.

[135] Griesser G (ed.) et al: Data Protection in health information systems. North Holland, 1980.

[136] Griesser G: Data Protection in Health Information Systems, MEDINFO 83: 950-953, North-Holland, 1983.

[137] Griesser G, Kenny D: Constructing guidelines for data protection in health information systems. MIE 79: 80-82, Springer-Verlag, 1979.

[146] Harding N: Data Protection in Medicine. TL Visuals, 1986.

[149] Hayes G: Data and Doctors. BJHC: 29, February 1989.

[221] Polter AR: Computers in general practice: the patient's voice. JRCGP **31**: 683-685, 1981.

[249] Rector Al, Sheldon MG: Privacy, data decay and the long term medical record. MIE 82: 686-691, Springer-Verlag, 1982.

[307] Thome R: Protection and Confidentiality of Medical Data - Efficient Data Protection through project specific combination of methods. MEDINFO 74: 189-191, Almqvist & Wiksell, 1974.

[312] Tsubo T: Safety and Security of Medical Information Systems. MEDINFO 80: 308-310, North-Holland, 1980.

[327] Williamson JD: Data protection and the clinician: guidelines on data security. BMJ **291**: 1516-1519, 1985.

[334] Anon: The Data Protection Act: more questions than answers. Practice Computing: 11-14, September, 1989.

[345] Anon: Ensuring that GPs can control confidentiality. Practice Computing: 16-17, Summer 1987.

[391] Anon: Confidentiality, records, and computers. BMJ **1**: 698-699, 1979.

[392] Anon: Computers and Confidentiality. BMJ **2**: 1663, 1978.

[393] Anon: Computers and Privacy. BMJ **1**: 178-179, 1976.

[394] Anon: Computers and Confidentiality in Medicine. (Conference Report from 27th WM Assy.). BMJ **4**: 290-292, 1973.

DIAGNOSIS / DECISION SUPPORT

[4]Adams ID et al: Computer-aided diagnosis of acute abdominal pain: a multicentre study. BMJ **293**: 800-804, 1986.

[10]Arborelius E, Timpka T: Study of the Practitioners' Knowledge Need and Use During Health Care Consultations: The Dilemma of the GP. MEDINFO 89: 101-105, North-Holland, 1989.

[29]Bassoe CF: A Combinatorial Diagnostic System for General Practice: Evaluation of the Social Impact of Disease by a Computerised Medical Record. MIE 88: 212-214, Springer-Verlag, 1988.

[31]Bavan N et al: Mickie - a microcomputer for medical interviewing. Int. J. of Man-Machine Studies **14**: 39-47, 1981.

[41]Borst F et al: MEDIAL: a natural language processing system for medical records. MIE 84: 128-133, Springer-Verlag, 1984.

[43]Bradshaw-Smith JH: Computer assisted screening effect on the patient and his consultation. BMJ **290**: 1709-1712, 1983.

[50]Brownbridge G et al: Effect of computer use in the consultation on the delivery of care. BMJ **291**: 639-642, 1985.

[53]Brownbridge G et al. The doctors use of a computer in the consulting room: an analysis. Int. J. Man-Machine Studies **21**: 65-90, 1984.

[56]Card WI, Lucas RW: Computer Interrogation in medical practice. Int. J. Man-Machine Studies **14**: 49-57, 1981.

[57]Carson NE, Oon YK: The computer in the consultation. J Fam Pract. **23**(5): 497-499, 1986.

[69]Croft DS: Is computerised diagnosis possible? Comp Bio Med Res **5**: 351 - 367, 1972.

212

[70]Cruickshank PJ: Computers in medicine: patients' attitudes. JRCGP **34**: 77-80, 1984.

[71]Cruickshank PJ: Patient Stress and the Computer in the Consulting Room. Social Science and Medicine **16**: 1371-1376, 1982.

[74]De Dombal FT et al: Simplified Computer-Aided Diagnosis of Acute Abdominal Pain. BMJ **2**: 73-75, 1975.

[75]De Dombal FT, Horrocks JC: Computer-aided Diagnosis: Conclusions from an overall Experience Involving 4469 patients. MEDINFO 74: 581-585, Almqvist & Wiksell, 1974.

[76]De Dombal FT et al: Human and Computer Aided Diagnosis of Abdominal Pain: Further report with emphasis on Performance of Clinicians. BMJ **1**: 376-380, 1974.

[77]De Dombal FT et al: Simulation of Clinical Diagnosis: A comparative study. BMJ **2**: 575-577, 1971.

[78]De Dombal FT et al: Computer aided Diagnosis of Acute Abdominal Pain. BMJ **2**: 9-13, 1972.

[79]De Dombal FT: Computer-Assisted Diagnosis of Abdominal Pain using "Estimates" Provided by Clinicians. BMJ **4**: 350-354, 1972.

[91]Difford F: Reducing Prescription Costs through computer controlled repeat prescribing. JRCGP **34**: 658-660, 1984.

[102] Dove G et al: General-practice history taking by computer: A "psychotropic" effect. MIE 79: 253-260. Springer-Verlag, 1979.

[103] Dove GA et al: The therapeutic effect of taking a patient's history by computer. JRCGP **27**: 477-481, 1977.

[104] Dove G, Norris P: Reflections on an interactive computerised history taking system in a general medical practice. MIE 82: 280-284, Springer-Verlag, 1982.

[109] Ellis D: Medical Computing and Applications. Ellis Harwood, 1987.

[119]Fox J, Alvey P: Computer assisted medical decision making. BMJ **287**: 742-745, 1983.

[154] Herzmark G et al: Consultation use of a computer by general practitioners. JRCGP **34**: 649-654, 1984.

[156] Hodgkin P: Reading the printout on the wall: decision making in general practice. BMJ **288**: 198-199, 1984.

[158] Horn W: ESDAT - Decision Support for primary medical care. MEDINFO 83: 484-487, North-Holland, 1983.

[159] Horrocks JC, De Dombal FT: Diagnosis of Dyspepsia from Data collected by a Physician's assistant. BMJ **3**: 421-423, 1975.

[160] Horrocks JC et al: Computer Aided Diagnosis: Description of an Adaptable System and Operational Experience with 2,034 cases. BMJ **2**: 5-9, 1972.

[167] Janecki J, Kokott H: Experiments with medical diagnostic systems. MIE 78: 29-36, Springer-Verlag, 1978.

[177] Kurashina S: Comparative Study of Computer-Aided Clinical Decision Making Systems. MEDINFO 80: 825-829, North-Holland, 1980.

[181] Leaper DJ et al: Clinical Diagnostic Process: An Analysis. BMJ **3**: 569-574, 1973.

[183] Limik B, Srdanovic V: An expert consultation system to aid clinical diagnoses. MIE 85: 138-142, Springer-Verlag, 1985.

[188] Lucas R et al: Computer Interrogation of Patients. BMJ **2**: 623-625, 1976.

[189] MacQueen D: Implications of primary health data capture. Current Perspectives in HC: 90-94, BJHC, 1988.

[206] Miller RA et al: INTERNIST-1 an experimental computer-based diagnostic consultant for general internal medicine. N.EngJMed **307**: 468-476, 1982.

[207] Miller RA et al: An experimental computer based diagnostic consultant for general internal medicine. N Eng J Med. **307**: 468 -478, 1982.

[211] Nilsson S et al: A computer in the physician's consultancy. MEDINFO 83: 1185-1186, North-Holland, 1983.

[218] Pelosi AJ, Lewis G: The computer will see you now. BMJ **299**: 138-139, 1989.

[228] Pringle M: Using Computers to take patient histories. BMJ **297**: 697, 1988.

[229] Pringle M et al: TIMER: a new objective measure of consultation content and its application to computer assisted consultations. BMJ **293**: 20-22, 1986.

[230] Pringle M et al: Topic analysis: an objective measure of the consultation and its application to computer assisted consultations. BMJ **290**: 1789-1791, 1988.

[233] Pritchard P: The information avalanche: can the GP survive. Practitioner **229**: 877-881, 1985.

[234] Pynsent PB, Fairback JC: Computer interview for patients with back pain. J. Biomed Eng II(1): 25-29, 1989.

[235] Quaak MJ: Comparison of data gathered with the help of an automated questionnaire and medical history data out of the medical record. MIE 85: 90-97, Springer-Verlag, 1985.

[236] Quaak MJ, Van der Voort PJ: Design of and experience with an automated questionnaire for medical history taking. MIE '84: 140-145, Springer-Verlag, 1984.

[237] Quaak MJ et al: Comparisons between written and computerised patient histories. BMJ **295**: 184-186, 1987.

[240] Rawlins D: Development of a family linkage program. Current Perspectives in HC: 31, BJHC, 1989.

[254] Reggia J: Computer Assisted Medical Decision Making. Springer-Verlag, 1985.

[255] Reggia JA, Tuhrim S (eds): Computer-assisted Decision Making. Springer-Verlag, 1985.

[257] Reichertz PL: Computer-Aided Medical Practice oriented towards diagnosis. MEDINFO 77: 191-197, North-Holland, 1977.

[262] Ridderkhoff J: Research into decision making strategies used in general practice. MIE 82: 272-279, Springer-Verlag, 1982.

[263] Ridderkhoff J: Diagnostic Decision Support System. MIE 87: 242, EDI Press, Rome, 1987.

[268] Roland M et al: Evaluation of a computer assisted repeat prescribing program in general practice. BMJ **291**: 456-458, 1985.

[272] Salaman R et al: Telematics & general practice: An experiment of a Drug Data Bank. MEDINFO 86: 246-248, North-Holland, 1986.

[277] Scadding JG: Diagnosis: the clinician and the computer. Lancet **2**: 877-881, 1967.

[292] Somerville S, et al: MICKIE - Experiences in taking histories from patients using a microcomputer. MIE 79: 713-721, Springer-Verlag, 1979.

[303] Taylor TR et al: Doctors as Decision Makers: A computer assisted study of diagnosis as a cognitive skill. BMJ **3**: 35-40, 1971.

[308] Timpka T: Introducing hypertext in primary health care: a study on the feasibility of decision support for practitioners. Comput Methods Programs Biomed **29**(1): 1-13, 1989.

[309] Timpka T et al: Decision Support for General Practitioners: Design and Implementation by Integrating Paradigms: Hypertext, Knowledge Based Systems and Online Library. MEDINFO 86: 96-100, North-Holland, 1986.

[310] Timpka T, Arborelius E: Study of the practitioner's knowledge need and use during health care consultations: Theory and Method. MEDINFO 89: 689-693, North-Holland, 1989.

[313] Tsumura H et al: Patient Oriented Multidisciplinary Medical Consultation System. MEDINFO 86: 289-293, North-Holland, 1986.

[325] White DH: The Computer Health Check - the first 100 patients. JRCGP **34**: 661-663, 1984.

[340] Anon: Screen Management: a view of the future? Practice Computing: 5-9, September 1988.

[356] Anon: Any Questions - computer interviewing. Practice Computing **12**(5): 18-19, October 1983.

[357] Anon: The Electronic Notebook. Practice Computing **2**(4): 18-20, 1983.

[382] Anon: A study of patients' attitudes to computer interrogation. Int. J. Man-Machine Studies **9**: 69-86.

[400] Anon: Knowledge-Based decision support for general practitioners: an integrated design. Computer Methods and Programs in Biomedicine **25**: 49-60, 1987.

PRESCRIBING

[15]Auvert B et al: Computer-Aided Prescription for General Practitioners using a hand held computer. MIE 85: 420-424, Springer-Verlag, 1985.

[16]Aylett M: Computerised repeat prescriptions: a simple system. BMJ **290**: 1115-1116, 1985.

[19]Bain DJ, Haines AJ: A year's study of drug prescription in general practice using computer-assisted records. JRCGP **25**: 41-48, 1975.

[32]BCS: A personal microcomputer data base in general practice. BCS - Primary Care Specialist Group Newsletter January 1987.

[38]Boon W, Molenaar RG: Medication Surveillance in Primary Health Care: Conditions for effectivity in an Information System for General Practice. MEDINFO 86: 254-258, North-Holland, 1986.

[49]Brown WD, Cordes DH: A microcomputer-assisted exercise prescription for use by family physicians. J Fam Pract. **27**(3): 267-270, 1988.

[94]Difford F et al: Maintaining the accuracy of a computer practice register: household index. BMJ **290**: 519-521, 1985.

[95]Difford F: Computer controlled repeat prescribing used to analyse drug management. BMJ **289**: 593-595, 1984.

[99]Donald JB: Prescribing costs when computers are used to issue all prescriptions. BMJ **299**: 28-30, 1989.

[100] Donald JB: On line prescribing by computer. BMJ **292**: 937-939, 1986.

[106] Ducrot H: Conditions of Use of Drug Information Systems designed for physicians or pharmacists. MEDINFO 83: 134, North-Holland, 1983.

[115] Fitter MJ, Garber R: (Repeat Prescription) - Is It Worth It? Practice Computing: **3**(3): 19-25, 1984.

[129] GMSC/RCGP Joint Computing Policy Group: BMJ **290**: 1252-1253, 1985.

[166] Irwin WG et al. Effect on prescribing of the limited list in a computerised group practice. BMJ **293**: 857-859, 1986.

[204] Meldrum D: Simple Computerised repeat prescription control system. BMJ **282**: 1933-1937, 1981.

[225] Preece JF et al: Writing all prescriptions by computer. JRCGP **34**: 655-657, 1984.

[239] Roschetti R: Prescription Monitoring System and Evaluation of Primary Care. MIE 87: 225-229, EDI Press , Rome, 1987.

[241] Rawson N, Inman W: Progress of a National Scheme for prescription-event monitoring in General Practice. MEDINFO 83: 141-144, North-Holland, 1983.

[266] Roberts D: Dispensing with computers: not an easy task. Practice Computing. 10-12, November 1989.

[295] Stevens R, Crabbe A: Experiences with Computer Card Medication Records in Britain. MIE 88: 180-184, Springer-Verlag, 1988.

[304] Telling JP et al: Developing a practice formulary as a by-product of computer controlled repeat prescribing. BMJ **288**: 1730-1732, 1984.

[361] Anon: Repeat Performer: (on repeat prescription systems). Practice Computing **2**(2): 18-23, 1983.

COMPUTERS IN GENERAL PRACTICE

[1] Abrams ME: Spectrum 71: A conference on Medical Computing.Oxford University Press, 1972.

[6]Akerman F M: Surgery computer - a quiet revolution for general practice. BMJ **288**: 1047-1053, 1984.

[10]Arborelius E, Timpka T: Study of the Practitioners' Knowledge Need and Use During Health Care Consultations: The Dilemma of the GP. MEDINFO 89: 101-105, North-Holland, 1989.

[11]Asbury AJ: To computerise or not. BMJ **286**: 2046-2049, 1982.

[13]Ashton JR: Micro Computers for general practitioners - an opportunity for collaboration. JRCGP **33**: 455-456, 1983.

[17]Aylett M: Advising GPs on IT. BJHC March 1988.

[18]Baharir Y, Epstein L: Computers in a community-oriented Practice of Family Medicine. MIE 88: 200-203, Springer-Verlag, 1988.

[21]Baldwin DW: Experience with micro computers in general practice. The Practitioner **229**: 643-646, 1985.

[22]Ball MJ, Snelbecker G: How physicians in the U.S. perceive computers in their practice. MEDINFO 83: 1169-1172, North-Holland, 1983.

[23]Banahan: Selecting a computer system for a medical practice. Prim Care **12**(3): 415-428, 1985.

[35]Billiet R, De Norre L: Comparative research, prevention and audit in general practice using the system oriented registration method. MIE 85: 368-372, Springer-Verlag, 1985.

[36]Billet R: System oriented registration in general practice.MIE 84: 546-551, Springer-Verlag, 1984.

[39]Boon WM, Duisterhart JS: ELIAS: Support for medical care. MEDINFO 89: 1205, North-Holland, 1989.

[42] Bozano P et al: An integrated development program in the field of primary care: the Ligurian Experience. MIE 87: 236-241, EDI Press, Rome, 1987.

[44] Bradshaw-Smith JH: The role of the computer in general practice. Practitioner **226:** 1211 - 1213, 1982.

[46] Brandejs JF, Pace GC: Physician's Primer on Computers. Lexington Books, 1979.

[48] Brown S: Views of general practitioners in the Oxford Region on microcomputing and collaboration with health authorities and family practitioner committees. JRCGP **38**: 115-116, 1988.

[51] Brownbridge G et al: An interactive computerised protocol for the management of hypertension: effects on the general practitioners' clinical behaviour. JRCGP **36**: 198-202, 1986.

[52] Brownbridge G et al: Patient Reactions to doctors' computer use in general practice consultations. Social Science & Medicine **20**: 47-52, 1985.

[59] Chan D et al: Implementation of a microcomputer-based opportunistic health maintenance programme in a general practice teaching clinic. Pulse: **47**(30): 1987.

[60] Chudley P: Putting a computer into practice has a rapid effect on patient care. Pulse: **47**(30): 1987.

[61] Clayton GM: Experience with an ICL 1905 Computer in General Practice. JRCGP **21**: 620-621, 1971.

[63] Cohen J: Computers in patient education. Postgrad Med **77**(4): 71-72, 1988.

[64] Coles E C: A Guide to Medical Computing. Butterworths, 1973.

[67] Covvey HD et al: Concepts and Issues in Health Care Computing. Mosby CV Company, 1985.

[81] De Moel J: General Practitioners' Information Systems: An Information System for Practice, Management, Research. MEDINFO 83, 1177-1180, North-Holland, 1983.

[82] De Moel J: General Practitioners Information System. MIE 82, 306-308, Springer-Verlag, 1982.

[86] DHSS: Survey of computerised general practices. NHS Info Tech Branch, 1987.

[87] DHSS: Joint Policy Computer Group. Micros in Practice: report of an appraisal of GP Micro Computer Systems. DHSS London HMSO, 1986.

[88] DHSS: Final Report. Project Evaluation Group. General Practice Computing - evaluation of the "Micro for GPs" scheme, London: HMSO, 1985.

[93] Difford F: Mapping practice population and morbidity with a computer. BMJ **291**: 1017-1020, 1985.

218

[94]Difford F et al: Maintaining the accuracy of a computer practice register: household index. BMJ **290**: 519-521, 1985.

[97]Dinwoodie HP, Howell RW: Automatic disease coding; the 'fruit machine' method in general practice. Br J Prev Soc Med **27** (1), 59 - 62, 1973.

[109] Ellis D: Medical Computing and Applications. Ellis Harwood, 1987.

[112] Fell PJ, Skees WD: The Doctor's Computer Handbook. Lifetime Learning Publications, 1984.

[114] Fitter MJ et al: A human factors evaluation of the IBM Sheffield Primary Care System. INTERACT **84**: 675 - 681, 1984.

[116] Fitter MJ: Making GP computers effective. BJHC: November 1986.

[117] Fitter MJ, Garber et al. (eds.): A Prescription for Change. - A report on the longer term use and development of computers in General Practice. London: HMSO, 1986.

[121] Gallen D: Don't buy a computer unless you research it. Financial Pulse, May 23 1989: 22-25.

[122] Gallen D: Practice progress: next create your own database. Financial Pulse, June 6, 1989: 35-36.

[123] Gallen D: Installation day ... the trials of the first weeks. Financial Pulse, June 20, 1989: 41.

[124] Gallen D: Theory to practice with our computers. Financial Pulse, August 15, 1989: 35.

[125] GMSC: Computers in General Practice. BMJ **280**: 662-663, 1980.

[126] GMSC: GMSC advises on computer contracts. BMJ **295**: 281, 1987.

[127] GMSC/RCGP Joint Computing Policy Group: 1982 Report. BMJ **286**: 660-661, 1983.

[132] Grace JF: A Computer in your practice: indispensable tool or troublesome toy? BMJ **285**: 1169-1171, 1982.

[134] Grene JD, Henderson JM: Automated recall in general practice. JRCGP **21**: 352-355, 1971.

[147] Hardy RH: Can I Computerise you now, Sir? JRCGP **15**: 233-237, 1968.

[148] Hargrave L et al: Computerised Family Practitioner Committee Records - a data base for general practice. JRCGP **38**: 22-23, 1988.

[152] Herd A: Multi - user systems: Panacea or pain in the neck? Practice Computing. 7 - 9, November 1989.

[157] Hogkinson M: Practice Computers. JRCGP **36**: 535, 1986.

[162] Howarth FP: Micros for GPs. BMJ **292**: 307-308, 1986.

[163] Howkins TJ, Kay CR: A computer-based appointment system for general practice. MEDINFO 89: 991-994, North-Holland, 1989.

[164] Hunday DS: Applications of personal computers in general practice. MIE 84: 565-566, Springer-Verlag, 1984.

[168] Jarman B: Giving advice about welfare benefits in general practice. BMJ **290**: 522-524, 1985.

[169] Jelovsek FR: Doctor's Office Computer Prep Kit. Springer Verlag, New York, 1985.

[171]Kay S, Davis R: How one GP computer system survived. Current Perspectives in HC: 148-154, BJHC, 1987.

[172] Kayll J: The computer key to information in general practice. Current Perspectives in HC: 37-48, BJHC, 1986.

[173] Keating J: GP acceptance of computer-generated hospital discharge letters. Current Perspectives in HC: 32, BJHC, 1989.

[182] Lewis A: Coming to terms with computers. Practitioner **231**: 1275 - 78, October 8th 1987.

[187] Lockley WJ: Mediscreen - a database for general practice. Current Perspectives in HC: 31-36, BJHC, 1986.

[190] Madeley RJ, Metcalfe DW: Doctors' attitudes to information systems - a survey of Derbyshire's general practitioners. JRCGP **28**: 654-658, 1978.

[191] Malcolm A, Poyser J: Computers and the General Practitioner (Proceedings of the GP-Info Symposium). London Pergamon Press, 1980.

[194] Marcus A: A plan for information in the National Health Service. Lancet **2**: 1242-1243, 1988.

[198] McCurry M: Microcomputers in General Practice - has there been any progress? Current Perspectives in HC: 65-73, BJHC, 1985.

[202] McWilliams A: Information technology in general practice. The Practitioner **231**: 1034 - 1037, 1987.

[205] Michel C et al: Validation of a Knowledge Base intended for General Practitioners to assist treatment of Diabetes: A blind study. MEDINFO 86: 122-127, North-Holland, 1986.

[209] Neal LR: The provision of data processing facilities for medical practitioners. MIE 78: 109-116, Springer-Verlag, 1978.

[211] Nilsson S et al: A computer in the physician's consultancy. MEDINFO 83: 1185-1186, North-Holland, 1978.

[213] Palmer P: Computing in General Practice. Scicon Consultancy International, 1980.

[220] Peumans W: Medical Computer Applications in Daily Practice by an Independent Group of Belgian Physicians. MEDINFO 74: 85-87, Almqvist & Wiksell, 1974.

[221] Polter AR: Computers in general practice: the patient's voice. JRCGP **31**: 683-685, 1981.

[222] Preece J: Are the GP system suppliers prepared? Practice Computing. 13 - 15, November 1989.

[223] Preece J: The use of computers in general practice. Churchill Livingstone, London, 1983.

[226] Pringle M: Using computers in general practice research. Practitioner **230:** 635 - 9, 1986.

[227] Pringle M: Greeks bearing gifts. BMJ **295:** 738 - 9, 1987.

[231] Pringle M et al: Computers in the surgery - the patient's view. BMJ **288:** 289-291, 1984.

[232] Pringle M et al: Computerisation: the choice. BMJ **284:** 165-168, 1982.

[233] Pritchard P: The information avalanche: can the GP survive. Practitioner **229:** 877-881, 1985.

[242] RCGP: Choosing a computer system. RCGP Members Reference Book, 1985.

[243] RCGP: Advice to members considering the current "no cost" computer systems. RCGP Publication, 1987.

[244] RCGP (Info Resources Centre): Computerising your practice. RCGP Publication, 1986.

[245] RCGP: Occasional Paper 13: Computers in Primary Care. Report of the Computer Working Party. RCGP Publication, 1980.

[247] Rector AL et al: A human computer interface for doctors. Current Perspectives in HC: 213-221, BJHC, 1988.

[253] Regester WD: The Physician's office system - How to maximise its use. MIE 84: 526-530, Springer-Verlag, 1984.

[256] Reichertz P, Schwarz B: Computers in the Doctor's Office: System Design, Physicians Motivation & Reaction. MEDINFO 80: 886-890, North-Holland, 1980.

[258] Reichertz PL et al: Results of a field test of computers for the private practice. MIE 79: 283-294, Springer-Verlag, 1979.

[265] Ritchie LD: Computers in Primary Care (Practicalities and Prospectus). Heinemann, London, 1984.

[271] Ryan MP: A national system for primary care computing. MEDINFO 89: 697-699, North-Holland, 1989.

[272] Salaman R et al: Telematics & general practice: An experiment of a Drug Data Bank. MEDINFO 86: 246-248, North-Holland, 1986.

[273] Salkind MR: Implementing a system in general practice. BMJ **287:** 199-201, 1983.

[274] Salkind MR: General Practice: Hardware & Software. BMJ **287:** 106-109, 1983.

[275] Saul PD: Accessing remote data bases using micro computers. JRCGP **35:** 384-386, 1985.

[276] Saunderson H: Potential benefits for patient care for computing. Community Medicine. **9** (3): 238 - 246, 1987.

[278] Scicon: Computers for General Practice: Conclusions of a feasibility study by Scicon Consultancy International. BMJ **2**: 884, 1980.

[279] Sheldon MG: The doctor, the patient and the computer. The Practitioner, **228**: 1121-1142, December, 1984.

[281] Sheldon MG: Satisfying the information needs of the general practitioner for improved patient care. MIE 78: 117-120, Springer-Verlag, 1978.

[282] Sheldon MG: Computers in General Practice: a personal view. JRCGP **34**: 647-648, 1984.

[293] South J: A computer summary used as a discharge letter. JRCGP **22**: 28-32, 1972.

[297] Stoddart N: The Computer in General Practice. The Practitioner **227**: 1825 - 1835, 1983.

[301] Symington et al: Shared-Care Project. Current Perspectives in HC: 19-21, BJHC, 1989.

[315] UpJohn Fellowship Report: Simple computer facilities in general practice. JRCGP: **19**: 269-281, 1970.

[323] Weeks R: For all those about to go online...... GP: August 21, 1987.

[326] Whitehouse CR: Preparing to introduce a computer into a Health Centre. BMJ **283**: 107-110, 1981.

[328] Willis A: GP Computer Systems. Pulse Reviews, 1987.

[330] Willis J: Bringing the visiting diary up to date. BMJ **292**: 1715-1716, 1986.

[335] Anon: Flying Start with a desktop network. Practice Computing: 19-20, February, 1989.

[341] Anon: Does a computerised practice make perfect? Practice Computing: 7-11, May 1988.

[342] Anon: Ten Questions for the free computer suppliers. Practice Computing Autumn 1987.

[343] Anon: Required reading for computer buyers. Practice Computing 1986 **4**(4): 26-27, February 1986.

[344] Anon: Reaping High Rewards (from an inexpensive system). Practice Computing **4**(4): 14-17, February 1988.

[346] Anon: Computerisation: A Methodical Approach. Practice Computing **4**(3): 4-7, 1985.

[348] Anon: A question of communication. Practice Computing: **4**(1): 8-12, 1985.

[350] Anon: Checklist for computing. Practice Computing Oct. 1984.

[351] Anon: A Tale of Two Systems. Practice Computing April 1984.

[352] Anon: Picking and Choosing (a system for a practice). Practice Computing: **3**(2): 6-8, 1984.

[355] Anon: How to live happily with a computer. Practice Computing :**2**(5): 20-22, 1983.

[358] Anon: The Next Step. Practice Computing: **2**(4): 11-12, 1983.

[362] Anon: Computers in Care: studying care for the chronically ill. Practice Computing:**1**(6): 18-21, 1982.

[365] Anon: Counting Costs - how much will a computer cost you? Practice Computing: **1**(4): 6-8, 1982.

[369] Anon: Practice buys into the computer age. Medeconomics: February 1989.

[370] Anon: Value for money is more than a big name. Medeconomics: January 1989.

[371] Anon: Get advice on making the most of a GP computer. Medeconomics: January 1988.

[372] Anon: Count costs to maintain your computer. Medeconomics: February 1987.

[373] Anon: Computers in Practice: 3 part series. Pulse April 1988.

[374] Anon: Evaluating medical computer systems. N.Z. Family Physician: Spring 1988.

[377] Anon: Computers in General Practice. Maternal and Child Health: 107, April 1989.

[381] Anon: Evaluating Feasibility and Selection of Computers in Family Medicine. Journal of Family Practice **19**(1): 86-92, 1984.

[383] Anon: GP Contract 1990 Survival Guide. GP: Nov/Dec. 1989.

[384] Anon: Taking the trauma out of a new practice computer. Financial Pulse **3**(21), 1988.

[386] Anon: Are you making the most of your practice computer? Financial Pulse **3**(6): 26 March, 1988.

[388] Anon: Free GP systems become comparable. BJHC **4** (5): 7, 1987.

[390] Anon: A computer in every surgery? BMJ **280**: 1556, 1980.

[399] Anon: A computer in the practice: Lessons learned in Sheffield. Computer Update: Autumn 1984.

[401] Anon: How to choose a general practice computing system: comparison of commercial packages. BMJ **297**: 838-840, 1988.

SCREENING / PREVENTION

[7]Ancill R et al: Screening for antenatal and postnatal depression symptoms in general practice using a microcomputer-delivered questionnaire. JRCGP **36**: 276-279, 1986.

[16]Aylett M: Computerised repeat prescriptions: a simple system. BMJ **290**: 1115-1116, 1985.

[18]Baharir Y, Epstein L: Computers in a community-oriented Practice of Family Medicine. MIE '88: 200-203, Springer-Verlag, 1988.

[27]Barber SG et al: System for long term review of patients at risk of becoming hyperthyroid. Lancet **2**: 967-967, 1977.

[28]Barnett GO et al: A computer-based monitoring system for follow-up of elevated blood pressure. Med Care 21(4): 400-409, 1983.

[33]Beilin LJ et al: Computer-Based Hypertension Clinic Records: A Co-operative Study. BMJ 2: 212,216, 1974.

[43]Bradshaw-Smith JH: Computer assisted screening effect on the patient and his consultation. BMJ **290**: 1709-1712, 1983.

[55]Bussey AL, Holmes BS: Immunisation levels - need they all decline? Lancet **2**: 970-971, 1977.

[59]Chan D et al: Implementation of a microcomputer-based opportunistic health maintenance programme in a general practice teaching clinic. Pulse: **47**(30): 1987.

[80]Degoulet P et al: Patient Compliance in hypertension care: the critical role of the computer. MIE 82: 288-295, Springer-Verlag, 1982.

[81]De Moel J: General Practitioners' Information Systems: An Information System for Practice, Management, Research. MEDINFO 83, 1177-1180, North-Holland, 1983.

[90]Difford F: A computerised audit of a screening programme to establish rubella immunity. JRCGP **36**: 371 - 372, 1986.

[92]Difford F et al: Continuous opportunistic and systematic screening for hypertension with computer help: analysis of non-responders. BMJ **294**: 1130-1132, 1987.

[94]Difford F et al: Maintaining the accuracy of a computer practice register: household index. BMJ **290**: 519-521, 1985.

[97]Dinwoodie HP, Howell RW: Automatic disease coding; the 'fruit machine' method in general practice. Br J Prev Soc Med **27** (1), 59 - 62, 1973.

[134] Grene JD, Henderson JM: Automated recall in general practice. JRCGP **21**: 352-355, 1971.

[150] Hedley A et al: Computer-assisted Follow Up Register for the NE of Scotland. BMJ **1**: 556-558, 1970.

[196] McAlister NH et al: Randomised Controlled trial of computer assisted management of hypertension in primary care. BMJ 293: 670-674, 1986.

[203] Meldrum D: Simple Computerised Disease Register. BMJ **282**: 191-194, 1981.

[214] Palombi L et al. A new system on a community oriented data base for the prevention of cardiovascular diseases in young people. MIE 87: 183-187, EDI Press, Rome, 1987.

[215] Pantin CFA, Merrett TG: Allergy screening using a micro-computer. BMJ **285**: 483-487.

[246] Read JD: Global Prevention in primary care - the GP's role. Current Perspectives in HC: 49, BJHC, 1986.

[260] Reynolds MT, Richards CW: Audit of computerised recall scheme for cervical cytology. BMJ **284**: 1375-1376, 1982.

[261] Richards B et al: A knowledge-based system for giving expert advice to the patient in all matters relating to conception, pregnancy and childbirth. MEDINFO 89: 1183, North-Holland, 1989.

[264] Rigby MJ: The National Child Health System In Practice. Current Perspectives in HC: 107-113, BJHC, 1987.

[269] Ronen I, Avitzour M: Computerisation of a Community Programme in Primary Health Care. MIE 87: 231-235, EDI Press, Rome, 1987.

[280] Sheldon MG: Using a micro-computer for doing monitoring in general practice. MIE 82: 380-386, Springer-Verlag, 1982.

[285] Shepherd SG: Comprehensive Preventative Medicine in General Practice: a new role for the micro computer. Current Perspectives in HC: 53-64, BJHC, 1989.

[289] Skinner HA et al: Lifestyle assessment: applying micro computers in family practice. BMJ **290**: 212-214, 1985.

[290] Smith C: Computer Programme to Estimate Recurrence Risks for Multifactorial Familial Disease. BMJ **1**: 495-497, 1972.

[291] Soljak MA, Handford S: Early results from the Northland immunisation register. NZ Med J **100**(822): 244-246, 1987.

[299] Sullivan D, Victor CR: Using computers for health education in general practice: a pilot study. Computers in Health Care Education and Training, 1988.

[311] Trower C: Data for Prevention - how GPs can do it. Current Perspectives in HC: 22-28, BJHC, 1988.

[316] Uplekor MW et al: Sympmed I: computer program for primary health care. BMJ **297**: 841-843, 1988.

[317] Vallbona C et al: Use of a computerised data base to monitor the level of control of hypertension in community health centres. MEDINFO 83: 261-264, North-Holland, 1983.

[324] Welch J: Computerised information retrieval services in a teaching hospital. BMJ **280**: 1433-1434, 1980.

[332] Anon: The impact of a micro computer on a practice immunisation clinic. The Practitioner **232**: 197, 1988.

[338] Anon: Health Screen - the only real cure is prevention. Practice Computing: 9-14, November 1988.

[339] Anon: Diabetes: rapid strides in computerised control. Practice Computing: 4-8, November 1988.

[398] Anon: A computer managed screening programme for the pre-symptomatic detection of cervical neoplasia. Current Perspectives in HC: 207-218, BJHC, 1984.

THE NHS, FPS AND THE GP

[1] Abrams ME: Spectrum 71: A conference on Medical Computing.Oxford University Press, 1972.

[3]Abrams ME: Health Services and the computer. Real time computing in general practice. Health Trends **4**: 18-20, 1972.

[14]Arnon PG et al: A computer communication network for hospitals and general practice. MEDINFO 89: 1121-1124, North-Holland, 1989.

[47]Brown J: Practicing EDT. BJHC: 27-28, February 1989.

[48]Brown S: Views of general practitioners in the Oxford Region on microcomputing and collaboration with health authorities and family practitioner committees. JRCGP **38**: 115-116, 1988.

[58]Cerutti S: The automatic treatment of the information in the medical records at the level of the general practitioner. MIE 82: 303-305, Springer-Verlag, 1982.

[73]Dean A: Developing the GP/FPC interface. Current Perspectives in HC : 29-34, 1988.

[84]Dezelic GJ et al: Development of health information systems for health centres delivering primary care in distributed environment. MIE 87, 203-208, EDI Press, Rome, 1987.

[85]Dezelic GJ et al: Development of a health data base for analysing the relation between environmental health and medical data with a micro computer. MIE 88: 185-189, Springer-Verlag, 1988.

[107] Duisterhout JS, Branger PJ: Communication in Primary Care Systems. MEDINFO 89: 700-703, North-Holland, 1989.

[113] Fisher RH: The role of FPS computing with regard to the problems of patient care computing as a whole. Current Perspectives in HC: 221-229, BJHC, 1984.

[138] Gruer KT: Livingstone New Town - Using a computer for general practice records. JRCGP **22**: 100-107, 1972.

[141] Hall J: A future strategy for FPS Computing. Current Perspectives in HC: 224-234, BJHC, 1985.

[142] Handby JG: Computerising Family Practitioner Services. MIE 85:373-379, Springer-Verlag, 1985.

[148] Hargrave L et al: Computerised Family Practitioner Committee Records - a data base for general practice. JRCGP **38**: 22-23, 1988.

[161] Houghton KA: Integrated data and opportunities for improving care. Current Perspectives in HC: 129-132, BJHC, 1987.

[173] Keating J: GP acceptance of computer-generated hospital discharge letters. Current Perspectives in HC: 32, BJHC, 1989.

[195] Masterman L: FPS Computerisation - the past, the present and the future. Current Perspectives in HC: 35, BJHC, 1989.

[197] McCurry MG: Large scale implementation of FPS computer systems in England and Wales. MIE 88: 473-477, Springer-Verlag, 1988.

[219] Petrie JC et al: Computer-assisted shared care in hypertension. BMJ **290:** 1960-1962, 1985.

[238] Rafanelli M et al: An integrated system for the general practitioner choice management. MIE 84: 552-557, Springer-Verlag, 1984.

[259] Renieri A: An information system for primary care (SIMB) as a link between local and national information systems. MIE 87: 613-620, EDI Press, Rome, 1987.

[264] Rigby MJ: The National Child Health System In Practice. Current Perspectives in HC: 107-113, BJHC, 1987.

[300] Sweeney J et al: Benefits of an integrated community system. Current Perspectives in HC: 122-128, BJHC, 1987.

[336] Anon: GP database - community resource. Practice Computing: 12-18, February 1989.

[337] Anon: Linking FPC and GP Systems. Practice Computing: 7-10, February 1989.

[379] Anon: Computerising FPC registers. JRCGP **32:** 67, 1982.

[397] Anon: IT for GPs. BJHC: 26-35, July 1988.

ADMINISTRATION / OFFICE AUTOMATION

[1] Abrams ME: Spectrum 71: A conference on Medical Computing. Oxford University Press, 1972.

[5] Ainslie J: Choosing a word processor. BMJ **298:** 514-515, 1989.

[12] Asbury AJ: Word Processing. BMJ **287:** 44-47, 1983.

[72] Day BD, Brandejs JF: Computers for Medical Office and Patient Management. Nostrand Reinhold, 1982.

[118] Fitter MJ et al: Computers and audit. JRCGP **35:** 522-524,1985.

[144] Hannaford PC, Hawkins TJ: Computer Support for Patient Management. Current Perspectives in HC: 85-89, BJHC, 1988.

[163] Howkins TJ, Kay CR: A computer-based appointment system for general practice. MEDINFO 89: 991-994, North-Holland, 1989.

[165] Ingram JA, Asbury AJ: Patient Administration - I/II. BMJ **287:** 600-603/667-670, 1983.

[174] Klaring WJ: CAPOS - Computer-aided physicians' office system. MIE 82: 285-287, Springer-Verlag, 1982.

[179] Law J: Manage to get the most from a computer. Medeconomics: December 1986.

[196] McAlister NH et al: Randomised Controlled trial of computer assisted management of hypertension in primary care. BMJ **293**: 670-674, 1986.

[208] Mohr J et al: Text Processing Systems for the doctors office. MIE 82: 262-271, Springer-Verlag, 1982.

[210] Nicholson WH, Canning B: The benefits of a patient administration system. Current Perspectives in HC: 165-169, BJHC, 1987.

[216] Payne JR, Hill DW (eds.): Real Time Computing in Patient Management. Peter Peregrines, 1975.

[270] Rothenberg LA, Aluise JJ: Implementing an automated financial management system for medical practices. J Fam Pract **18**(5): 785-790, 1984.

[298] Studin JR, Kalisman M: Computers and Medical Office Management. Clin Plast Surg **13**(3): 367-374, 1986.

[363] Anon: Computer Manager. Practice Computing **1**(5): 22-23, 1982.

[385] Anon: Learning how to manage computerised accounts. Financial Pulse: 23 April 1988.

ADVANCES / DEVELOPMENTS / TRENDS

[34]Bennett WL: The Computer and the Clinician. MEDINFO 74: 133-136, Almqvist & Wiksell, 1974.

[37]BMA: Computers in Medicine. BMA Planning Unit: Report No. 3, 1969.

[65]Coleridge Smith PD, Scurr JH (eds.): Medical Applications of Microcomputers. Springer-Verlag, 1988.

[67]Covvey HD et al: Concepts and Issues in Health Care Computing. 1985.

[83]Dezelic GJ et al: Computer Assisted Instruction in Continuing Education for Primary Health Care: Project Concepts and Development. MEDINFO 89, 1078-1082, North-Holland, 1989.

[89]Difford F: Future trends in general practice computing. JRCGP **37**: 434-435, 1987.

[109] Ellis D: Medical Computing and Applications. Ellis Harwood, 1987.

[127] GMSC/RCGP Joint Computing Policy Group: 1982 Report. BMJ **286**: 660-661, 1983.

[128] GMSC/RCGP Joint Policy Computing Group: 1983 Report. BMJ **289**: 1242, 1984.

[130] GMSC/RCGP Joint Computing Policy Group: Standards for computer issued prescriptions. Research and Development in Primary Care computing. JRCGP **32**: 88-92, 1982.

[131] GMSC/RCGP Joint Policy Computing Group: General Practice Report for 1981. JRCGP **32**: 197-198, 1982.

[140] Gunner C: The implications of smart card technology. Current Perspectives in HC: 236-240, BJHC, 1988.

[143] Handby JG: Harnessing Technology to health care - the challenge for the future. MIE 84: 616-621, Springer-Verlag, 1984.

[170] Johnson RA: Computer analysis of the complete medical record including symptoms and treatment. JRCGP **22**: 655-660, 1972.

[193] Mann N: Smart Cards in Health Care: A solution in search of a problem. MEDINFO '89: 1151-1155, North-Holland, 1989.

[200] McLachlan G, Shegog RR: Computers in the Service of Medicine. London Oxford University Press, 1968.

[201] McWilliams A: The age of the computer. JRCGP **36** (292): 490 - 491, 1986.

[212] Ockenden J, Bodenhamp: Focus on Medical Computer Development. OUP, 1970.

[217] Payne LC, Brown PT: An introduction to medical automation, Pitman Medical, London, 1975.

[245] RCGP: Occasional Paper 13: Computers in Primary Care. Report of the Computer Working Party. RCGP Publication, 1980.

[265] Ritchie LD: Computers in Primary Care (Practicalities and Prospectus). Heinemann, London, 1984.

[267] Robinson ND: General practice - a technological future. The Practitioner **230**: 867, 1986.

[271] Ryan MP: A national system for primary care computing. MEDINFO 89: 697-699, North-Holland, 1989.

[279] Sheldon MG: The doctor, the patient and the computer. The Practitioner, **228**: 1121-1142, December, 1984.

[284] Sheldon M, Stoddard N: Trends in General Practice Computing. RCGP, 1985.

[286] Shortliffe E, Claney W: Readings in Medical Artificial Intelligence: the first decade. Addison-Wesley, 1984.

[302] Tanner S: Expert Systems: starting small. Practice Computing :5(9), 1987.

[314] Turner RD et al: Computers in primary care: where next? BMJ 2: 1020-1022, 1980.

[320] Vohloren I: Measurement of Productivity in Primary Care. MIE 85: 399-403, Springer-Verlag, 1985.

[321] Walker CH: "Batch" or "on-line" for child health - a review. BMJ **281**: 90-92, 1980.

[329] Willis A, Stewart T: Computers: A Guide to Choosing and Using. Oxford University Press, 1989.

[331] Young DW: A survey of decision aids for clinicians. BMJ **285**: 1332-1335, 1982.

[333] Anon: The long road to Government funding of GP systems. Practice Computing: 8-10, September 1989.

[342] Anon: Ten Questions for the free computer suppliers. Practice Computing Autumn 1987.

[347] Anon: A Stand on Standards. Practice Computing: **4**(2): 5-7, 1985.

[349] Anon: A quite bright future. Practice Computing December 1984.

[354] Anon: Computers in Perspective. Practice Computing: **3**(1): 16-17, 1984.

[359] Anon: Computer Forum 1. Forum between RCGP and BCS. Practice Computing: **2**(3): 8-13, 1983.

[360] Anon: Past, Present and Future. (History and development of Practice Systems). Practice Computing: **2**(2): 24-25, 1983.

[364] Anon: Where do we go from here? the next step for computing in general practice. Practice Computing: **1**(5): 19-21, 1982.

[366] Anon: High tech response to a new NHS hits obstacles. Medeconomics: July 1989.

[367] Anon: The future of GP computing is taking shape now. Medeconomics: May 1989.

[368] Anon: Computer suppliers vie for GPs custom. Medeconomics: March 1989.

[375] Anon: Introducing expert systems to medical students using ESTA, Expert System Teaching Aid. Medical Education **22**: 99-103, 1988.

[376] Anon: Computerisation in primary health care. The Medical Annual: 1986.

[378] Anon: Why doctors don't use computers: some empirical findings. J. Royal Society of Medicine **79**: 1986.

[380] Anon: Computers in Primary Care. JRCGP **30**: 387-388, 1980.

[389] Anon: Computers in medicine: searching for the rainbow and the crock of gold. BMJ **284**: 1859-1860, 1982.

[395] Anon: Expert Systems. BJHC: 40, January 1986.

[396] Anon: Scottish Health Computing. BJHC: January 1986.

FULL REFERENCES INDEX

[1]   Abrams ME: Spectrum 71: A conference on Medical Computing.
Oxford University Press, 1972.
E/H/G
The text consists of papers given at the conference by various experts. It sets out to be a platform for discussion by those looking to use computers in the NHS environment. Many of the papers are applicable (directly) to primary care. There are chapters on doctor/patient relationships, general practice administration and long range planning.

[2]Abrams ME: Computer terminals in a health centre. Community Health
   3: 81-85, 1971.

A
A research project with the aim of establishing whether an integrated records system will help improve the practice of medicine and the standard of patient care in the community, and at an acceptable cost. The article looks at facilities available and problems with the system.

[3]Abrams ME: Health Services and the computer. Real time computing in
   general practice. Health Trends **4**: 18-20, 1972.
A/G
In the development of medical services for Thamesmead (a New Town) it rapidly became apparent, when discussing the medical record system that would be needed, that a properly integrated record system would be necessary. This article describes the benefits of the system and the use of the computer in the system.

[4]Adams ID et al: Computer-aided diagnosis of acute abdominal pain: a
   multicentre study. BMJ **293**: 800-804, 1986.

C
A multicentre study of computer aided diagnosis for patients with acute abdominal pain was performed in 8 centres with over 250 participating doctors and 16737 patients. The study concludes computer aided diagnosis is a useful system for improving diagnosis and encouraging better clinical practice.

[5]Ainslie J: Choosing a word processor. BMJ **298**: 514-515, 1989.

H
Before rushing out to buy a word processor perhaps you should ask why you are parting with your money.

[6]Akerman F M: Surgery computer - a quiet revolution for general
   practice. BMJ **288**: 1047-1053, 1984.

E
This paper shows how computerisation can transform a practice's programme of prevention and surveillance. It discusses the initial hostility of staff and shows how the computer became accepted and played an important role in office efficiency and accuracy. It shows how results in a range of surveillance and prevention areas have improved.

[7]Ancill R et al: Screening for antenatal and postnatal depression symptoms in general practice using a microcomputer-delivered questionnaire. JRCGP **36**: 276-279, 1986.

F

The study screened 108 women throughout pregnancy and trends were observed and analyses made. The routine use of microcomputers to administer questionnaires to patients has proved feasible within general practice.

[8]Anderson J: Clinical Records System: An Overview. Current Perspectives in HC. 107-114, BJHC,1984.

A

Clinical records are an essential part of health care, both in the immediate situation and for control and guidance. They are at the base of any care system. Only with better computerised clinical information systems is it going to be possible to guide and control the delivery of optimal health care in a world of competing resources.

[9] Anderson J, Forsythe J: Information Processing of Medical Records. North-Holland, 1970.

A

A collection of papers presented at a conference "The Information Processing of Medical Records" which covers all areas in vogue at the time, including development of systems, questionnaires, linkage processing, and validation of medical records.

[10]   Arborelius E, Timpka T: Study of the Practitioners' Knowledge Need and Use During Health Care Consultations: The Dilemma of the GP. MEDINFO **89**: 101-105, North-Holland,1989.

C/E

For system development, a study of problems faced by GPs during consultations was made. From 46 consultations by 12 GPs, 262 'dilemmas' were recorded. Implications for design of computer-based decision support systems and continued medical education are discussed. The method used in the study showed to obtain a unique set of data, essential for system development involving consultation situations.

[11]   Asbury AJ: To computerise or not. BMJ **286**: 2046-2049, 1982.

E

The article describes the steps of implementing a computer in a small business. It is important to remember than a computer is not a panacea; it will not produce efficiency where the practice on which it is based is not efficient. In some cases the improved organisation which computer use imposes produces a greater improvement in efficiency than the computer. In even the simplest case where a microcomputer is being considered much thought must be given to matching the computer to the task.

[12]   Asbury AJ: Word Processing. BMJ **287**: 44-47, 1983.

H

Word processing can be of help to all types of doctor e.g. the general practitioner who would like to speed up production of referral letters. This article looks at what facilities are available.

[13]   Ashton JR: Micro Computers for general practitioners - an opportunity for collaboration. JRCGP **33**: 455-456, 1983.

E

For the adoption of computers to be justified it should be possible to demonstrate improved efficiency and effectiveness for the work being carried out; and for this to be possible objectives need to be stated and made explicit, and outcome measures must be developed.

[14]   Arnon PG et al: A computer communication network for hospitals and general practice. MEDINFO 89: 1121-1124, North-Holland, 1989.

G

In this paper the position of general practitioners in Dutch Health Care and the benefits of using a computer communication network between hospitals and general practice are discussed. Also the development of the network is described. Technical details of the network and the use of Electronic Data Interchange in health care computer communications are mentioned.

[15]   Auvert B et al: Computer-Aided Prescription for General Practitioners using a hand held computer. MIE 85: 420-424, Springer-Verlag, 1985.

D

A description of the PHARMAID system, and the software and hardware of which it comprises. This is followed by a discussion of the future of such hand-held systems in medicine, the very wide usage expected within 10 years, and why it is that they are complementary with telematic information networks.

[16]   Aylett M: Computerised repeat prescriptions: a simple system. BMJ **290**: 1115-1116, 1985.

D/F

A program that can maintain a patient register, check mileage and dispensing figures, prepare call-up lists for inoculations, search specific age groups for particular conditions, as well as provide a repeat prescription function, is described.

[17]   Aylett M: Advising GPs on IT. BJHC March 1988.

E

A report which says that if general practice computing is to progress, regional advisors should be appointed.

[18]   Baharir Y, Epstein L: Computers in a community-oriented Practice of Family Medicine. MIE 88: 200-203, Springer-Verlag, 1988.

E/F

The major principle of governing the delivery of community oriented Primary Health Care is the provision of comprehensive health and medical care in relation to the epidemiologically determined needs of the community. For this the practice team requires data related to both population and its health needs. This report looks at computers being used in this role.

[19]   Bain DJ, Haines AJ: A year's study of drug prescription in general practice using computer-assisted records. JRCGP **25**: 41-48, 1975.

D

In a practice the records were computerised; some of the problems involved are mentioned. The lessons to be learnt from self audit have been shown and areas for future study are discussed.

[20]   Bakker A, Louwese C: Considerations on the Effectiveness of
         Protection by Passwords. MIE 85: 343-346, Springer-Verlag, 1985.

B

This article looks at the two ways a password can be used - computer generated and user supplied - and analyses the vulnerability and guess-risk of each method. It also suggests ways in which the vulnerability of passwords can be reduced.

[21]   Baldwin DW: Experience with micro computers in general practice.
         The Practitioner **229**: 643-646, 1985.

E

The micro computer is not receiving a totally enthusiastic welcome in general practice judging from the results of a survey among practices using this machine in Lancashire and Yorkshire. Nevertheless, the author feels optimistic about its potential, given the inadequacy of the present record keeping systems.

[22]   Ball MJ, Snelbecker G: How physicians in the U.S. perceive
         computers in their practice. MEDINFO 83: 1169-1172, North-Holland,
         1983.

E

As physicians become more computer literature they have more input into deciding where and how computers should be used. So it becomes increasingly important to obtain physicians' views on computer technology to improve patient care. This study assesses and collects empirical data on the subject.

[23]   Banahan: Selecting a computer system for a medical practice. Prim
         Care **12**(3): 415-428, 1985.

E

The risk of selecting an inadequate computer for a practice can be minimised when the selection process is done properly. A seven-step approach for selecting an office management system is described, with discussion of major factors to consider and pitfalls to avoid.

[24]   Barber B: Getting Our DP act together. BJHC **4** (5): 32-36, 1987.

B This article sets out the hurdles that have to be overcome quickly by the NHS in order to comply with the Data Protection Act which is to come into effect by 11 November 1987.

[25]   Barber B: Wanted: A Confidentiality Clause in Staff Contracts. BMJ **2**:
         702, 1973.

B

The introduction of computers has highlighted issues concerning confidentiality but do not themselves increase or decrease the level of confidentiality. This article points out where the responsibilities lie and addresses some key points of the program.

[26]   Barber JH: Computer assisted recording in general practice. JRCGP **21**: 726 - 736, 1971.

A General practice in Livingstone New Town is concerned with two major experiments the fusion of hospital, local authority, and general practice, in a unified health service and the application of computer techniques to practice recording. This paper describes the computer output for the year 1970 in respect of one of the Livingstone practices.

[27]   Barber SG et al: System for long term review of patients at risk of becoming hyperthyroid. Lancet **2**: 967-967, 1977.

F

Eight years experience of a computer assisted system for long term follow-up of patients at risk of hyperthyroidism shows that the system is reliable, efficient, and economical.

[28]   Barnett GO et al: A computer-based monitoring system for follow-up of elevated blood pressure. Med Care **21**(4): 400-409, 1983.

F

An automated surveillance system utilising a computer-based medical record system (COSTAR) was designed to improve the follow-up of patients with newly identified elevated diastolic blood pressure. This study concludes that a computer-based reminder system improves follow-up of newly discovered elevation in diastolic blood pressure.

[29]   Bassoe CF: A Combinatorial Diagnostic System for General Practice: Evaluation of the Social Impact of Disease by a Computerised Medical Record. MIE 88: 212-214, Springer-Verlag, 1988.

A/C

A general problem solving method has been tested using a computerised medical record. Present findings indicate that the combinatorial diagnostic process may well facilitate the study of single causes of disease even if the context is complex. In addition, the method is suitable for a practice computer.

[30]   Bassoe C, Sorli W: A Problem-Oriented Computerised Medical Record worked whereas a Chronological did not. MIE 88: 190-199, Springer-Verlag, 1988.

A

A chronological computerised medical record, within 3 years, ran into problems requiring time consuming editing to elicit suitable information. PROMED was developed to overcome these problems, allowing rapid switching between problems and sorting of data, etc. The paper concludes that computerised medical records require a problem-oriented approach.

[31]   Bavan N et al: Mickie - a microcomputer for medical interviewing. Int. J. of Man-Machine Studies **14**: 39-47, 1981.

C
A system has been developed for taking medical histories, by microcomputer, from patients. The doctor specifies the interview in the form of a numbered flow-chart. When presented to the patient this emulates a friendly doctor asking questions requiring simple yes/no answers. The system is easy to use and collects accurate information.

[32]   BCS: A personal microcomputer data base in general practice. BCS - Primary Care Specialist Group Newsletter January 1987.

D
A database program on a micro-computer was used to store details of patients who frequently visited the doctor. The information was used for repeat prescriptions, printing treatment labels, and monitoring patients needing regular attention.

[33]   Beilin LJ et al: Computer-Based Hypertension Clinic Records: A Co-operative Study. BMJ **2**: 212,216, 1974.

A/F
A computer based medical record system has been developed to help with research into hypertension and the management of patients with hypertension. Standard medical records are replaced by data collection forms, and case-notes are printed by the computer. A document which is generated for recording information at follow-up visits contains an up-to-date summary of the important clinical features with warnings of risk factors. A blood-pressure graph and a letter for the GP are produced on request.

[34]   Bennett WL: The Computer and the Clinician. MEDINFO 74: 133-136, Almqvist & Wiksell, 1974.

I
A look at present trends, potentials, and future objectives of computers in clinical practice.

[35]   Billiet R, De Norre L: Comparative research, prevention and audit in general practice using the system oriented registration method. MIE 85: 368-372, Springer-Verlag, 1985.

A/E
An automated, practice-size denominator is presented. Research and audit are possible not only within one practice but also between different practices. Of all the monitored parameters, the statistical results of the search can be presented in graphic and synoptic print-outs. The Minimum Basic Data Set can be realised on the general practice level. Some of the possibilities of using an automated medical record system are emphasised.

[36]   Billet R: System oriented registration in general practice. MIE 84: 546-551, Springer-Verlag, 1984.

A/E
Registration of data relative to the patient can be achieved by different methods. The paper presents a method with its starting point in the Problem Oriented Medical Record System (Weed, 1969). The aim was to automate, as far as possible, the efficient registration of all data, the supervision of all files, the use of recall facilities, and to perform the secretarial as well as the book-keeping work. The possibility to do practice surveys (optimise the

comparability of patient-data and to enable comparative research between different practices) was looked for.

[37]   BMA: Computers in Medicine. BMA Planning Unit: Report No. 3, 1969.

I

Written when computers were still very new in medicine, the report addresses issues concerning ethics and future development, and calls attention to the difficult relationship that arises between Government and the Health Service. The report aims to be a reliable primer for the use of doctors.

[38]   Boon W, Molenaar RG: Medication Surveillance in Primary Health Care: Conditions for effectivity in an Information System for General Practice. MEDINFO 86: 254-258, North-Holland, 1986.

It is clear that medication surveillance (prescription control) should take place in general practice, not only in pharmacies. Arguments in favour of this, and the pitfalls, are presented here. To create an optimal drug surveillance system, with minimal false-positive or false-negative messages, extra information needs to be added to the commonly used drug and diagnosis data bases. This paper highlights the conditions the different data bases must meet, and suggests what supplementary information is needed.

[39]   Boon WM, Duisterhart JS: ELIAS: Support for medical care. MEDINFO 89: 1205, North-Holland, 1989.

E

A short comment on the ELIAS system, used in general practice in the Netherlands, and the uses and advantages of such an information system.

[40]   Borque M et al: Access to a medical advice and referral system: Avoiding the Chinese Menu System. MEDINFO 86: 282-284, North-Holland, 1986.

C

Dr. Oncall is a computer-based medical advice and referral system addressing over 100 signs and symptoms. The design is geared towards consultation through public access stations. This paper describes a simple effective access module that was developed on the basis of numeric input through a ruggedized keypad.

[41]   Borst F et al: MEDIAL: a natural language processing system for medical records. MIE 84: 128-133, Springer-Verlag, 1984.

A

This paper presents an experimental system for on-line analysis of medical records. It is intended to overcome the traditional conflict between processing requirements (i.e. fixed standardised data) and users' needs (i.e. free text). An overview of MEDIAL (MEdical DIALogues) is given.

[42]   Bozano P et al: An integrated development program in the field of primary care: the Ligurian Experience. MIE 87: 236-241, EDI Press, Rome, 1987.

E

This experiment has four main aims: i) the installation of a microcomputer into the booking centres office; ii) the distribution of a magnetic badge for health identity; iii) the installation of a personal computer into GP's surgeries; iv) the evaluation of the usefulness of data provided by GPs. The paper describes the system and details the experimental evaluation.

[43]   Bradshaw-Smith JH: Computer assisted screening effect on the patient and his consultation. BMJ **290**: 1709-1712, 1983.

C/F

The initial impact of computer assisted preventative screening in general practice consultations has been monitored. This article reports on the conclusions and results.

[44]   Bradshaw-Smith JH: The role of the computer in general practice. Practitioner **226**: 1211 - 1213, 1982.

E The author looks at the computer in the role of managing the practice and looks at ways in which the computer is applied. Some of the mystic surrounding computers is dispelled. Some advantages and disadvantages are discussed.

[45]   Bradshaw-Smith JH: A computer record-keeping system for general practice. BMJ **1**: 1395-1397, 1976.

A

In 1970 Preece showed the feasibility of keeping general practice records on computer. In 1975 the Ottery St. Mary practice started using a real time computer maintained record to replace the NHS envelope. This paper describes the record and the way it was used.

[46]   Brandejs JF, Pace GC: Physician's Primer on Computers. Lexington Books, 1979.

E

The book is aimed at physicians in practice who are looking to improve their practices. The book explains how this can be accomplished through the implementation of a modern computer/communications technology. The book uses a minimum of jargon and can be understood by those with no computer experience.

[47]   Brown J: Practicing EDT. BJHC: 27-28, February 1989.

G

A description of a trial experimenting with electronic data transfer (EDT), sending patient registration details from the practice to FPC by computer links.

[48]   Brown S: Views of general practitioners in the Oxford Region on microcomputing and collaboration with health authorities and family practitioner committees. JRCGP **38**: 115-116, 1988.

E/G

The results of a postal questionnaire to investigate interest in microcomputing and in pooling data with other health authorities and FPCs.

[49]   Brown WD, Cordes DH: A microcomputer-assisted exercise prescription for use by family physicians. J Fam Pract. **27**(3): 267-270, 1988.

D

Family physicians frequently advise their patients on choosing and implementing regular programmes of exercise. The report describes techniques of submaximal aerobic fitness assessment and microcomputer-assisted exercise prescription suitable for use in office-based practices. This approach is practical for young to middle-aged low-risk individuals interested in beginning regular training programmes.

[50]   Brownbridge G et al: Effect of computer use in the consultation on the delivery of care. BMJ **291**: 639-642, 1985.

C

In this trial, a computer system provided for the review and update of patients' medical histories, on doctor-patient contacts, and information on repeat prescribing. Consultations in which no computer was used are compared.

[51]   Brownbridge G et al: An interactive computerised protocol for the management of hypertension: effects on the general practitioners' clinical behaviour. JRCGP **36**: 198-202, 1986.

E

This paper focuses particularly on the protocol's effect on doctors' clinical behaviour. The computerised protocol is compared to the original paper based version. Doctors delivery of care was assessed.

[52]   Brownbridge G et al: Patient Reactions to doctors' computer use in general practice consultations. Social Science & Medicine **20**: 47-52, 1985.

E

This paper describes an experimental field study of patient reactions to computer use by doctors during general practice consultations. The computer system offered facilities for the review of medical industries and the entry of individual encounter notes. Questionnaire assessments of patient reactions were obtained from 127 patients who had just consulted a doctor who was using the computer, and from 216 control patients for whom conventional procedures remained. Results suggest the reaction of patients has more to do with which doctor they see than whether they use a computer.

[53]   Brownbridge G et al. The doctors use of a computer in the consulting room: an analysis. Int. J. Man-Machine Studies **21**: 65-90, 1984.

C

A human factors assessment of an interactive computer-aid to history-taking and diagnosis. Monitoring consultations before and after the computer's installation enabled an assessment of the computer's influence on the doctors' information gathering and processing.

[54]   Bulpitt CJ et al. Randomised controlled trial of computer-held medical records in hypertensive patients. BMJ **1**: 677-679, 1976.

A

A total of 278 hypertensive patients were allocated to either have their medical records held on computer or on standard hospital notes. For the computer system doctors completed a structured input form, and symptoms, physical findings, and diagnoses were more complete than on hospital notes. The paper also draws conclusions on clinic management and effects on patient care and management.

[55]   Bussey AL, Holmes BS: Immunisation levels - need they all decline?
         Lancet **2**: 970-971, 1977.

F

Immunisation levels of certain illnesses did not reflect the national average in West Sussex, which showed a better record of vaccinations. It is suggested that this difference is accounted for by the use of a computer system which keeps an immunisation diary for parents and medical staff.

[56]   Card WI, Lucas RW: Computer Interrogation in medical practice. Int.
         J. Man-Machine Studies **14**: 49-57, 1981.

C

This paper describes the examination of the possibility of using computer interrogation in this country, the position which the technique has reached today, and the possible future envisaged for it.

[57]   Carson NE, Oon YK: The computer in the consultation. J Fam Pract.
         23(5): 497-499, 1986.

C

This paper briefly outlines a development in the area of patient care applications. The authors do not consider the computer a too distant consultant, but one capable of improving patient care. The systems will need to provide high-speed response, multi-tasking including interrupt ability, and a range of imaginative modules integrated with a flexible and transportable medical record.

[58]   Cerutti S: The automatic treatment of the information in the medical
         records at the level of the general practitioner. MIE 82: 303-305,
         Springer-Verlag, 1982.

A/G

This paper looks at research being carried out in Italy aiming at the definition, the analysis, and the implementation of an operation system, for the collection and the distribution of the information at the various levels of health operators, and hence, even at GPs.

[59]   Chan D et al: Implementation of a microcomputer-based opportunistic
         health maintenance programme in a general practice teaching clinic.
         Pulse: **47**(30): 1987.

E/F

A set of protocols has been written for a list of health maintenance items and a computer has been programmed to identify items which should be carried out at each patient encounter in order to implement a uniform and up-to-date health maintenance programme.

[60]   Chudley P: Putting a computer into practice has a rapid effect on
         patient care. Pulse: **47**(30): 1987.

E

A description of how a Solihull practice has boosted immunisation and screening using a computer, and recognises that GPs who computerise purely to maximise income could be disappointed.

[61]   Clayton GM: Experience with an ICL 1905 Computer in General Practice. JRCGP **21**: 620-621, 1971.

E

A short description of the development of a very simple system for register maintenance in general practice using an ICL 1905 computer.

[62]   Cobbs JS, Miles DP: Estimating list inflation in a practice register. BMJ **287**: 1434-1436, 1983.

A

The reasons why patients were incorrectly registered in an age-sex register were studied, and under-registration was found due to delay in registration administration. It is suggested that a computer package in general practice could correct the population size and structure for estimated list inflation.

[63]   Cohen J: Computers in patient education. Postgrad Med **77**(4): 71-72, 1988.

E

The author offers guidance on selecting a computerised patient-education system and installing it in your practice.

[64]   Coles EC: A Guide to Medical Computing. Butterworths, 1973.

E

A specialist monograph providing a simple introduction to the hardware and software of computers together with a useful glossary of terms. It should supply valuable background information to doctors new to computing techniques but who need to make use of them in their work.

[65]   Coleridge Smith PD, Scurr JH (eds.): Medical Applications of Microcomputers. Springer-Verlag, 1988.

I

Deals with microcomputer applications in a wide area of clinical applications including discussion of recent developments in several clinical specialities.

[66]   Cormack J: The General Practitioners Use of Medical Records. Edinburgh University, 1970.

A

A medical thesis based on the hypothesis that conventional record keeping systems are inadequate. The thesis discusses the application of computers to medical record keeping.

[67]   Covvey HD et al: Concepts and Issues in Health Care Computing. Mosby CV Company,1985.

E/I

Having acknowledged the importance and pervasiveness of computer technology, the book sets about demystifying the technology. It is also written as an aid to health care professionals in identifying the limitations and use of computers. The book approaches the communication problem between health care professionals and computer professionals in order to increase the computer competence of the health care professionals.

[68]   Crambie DL: Record linkage in automated systems. JRCGP **31**: 325-326, 1981.

A/B
A look at the advantages, problems and confidentiality of automated records.

[69]   Croft DS: Is computerised diagnosis possible? Comp Bio Med Res **5**: 351 - 367, 1972.

C A look at the "real" problems of practical computer aided diagnosis i.e, (1) lack of standard medical definitions, (2) lack of large reliable medical databases and (3) lack of acceptance of computer-aided diagnosis by the medical profession. The author suggests the formation of a liaison group.

[70]   Cruickshank PJ: Computers in medicine: patients' attitudes. JRCGP **34**: 77-80, 1984.

C
Two surveys measured patients attitudes to diagnostic computers and medical computers in general. Among others, a notable finding was that over half the group believed that, with a computer around, the personal touch of the doctor would be lost.

[71]   Cruickshank PJ: Patient Stress and the Computer in the Consulting Room. Social Science and Medicine **16**: 1371-1376, 1982.

C
This study assesses patient reactions to the use of diagnostic computers by doctors. Patient reactions were measured through a mixed questionnaire of stress and arousal and a questionnaire on the medical use of computers. It is suggested that doctors planning to use computers should take care to preserve their human touch particularly for nervous patients.

[72]   Day BD, Brandejs JF: Computers for Medical Office and Patient Management. Nostrand Reinhold, 1982.

H
This book provides an up-to-date coverage of computers for computing health data and mapping disease and environmental data. The book provides strategies for keeping costs down and improving inter-disciplinary communication. Computer systems currently on the market are examined by experts to provide a good guide to the ability of the computers.

[73]   Dean A: Developing the GP/FPC interface. Current Perspectives in HC : 29-34, BJHC, 1988.

G
Such an interface would provide faster, easier transfer of data; more efficient services to GPs; more efficient FPCs; but, fundamentally better patient care; to use the resources and facilities of FPCs and GPs to best effect.

[74]   De Dombal FT et al: Simplified Computer-Aided Diagnosis of Acute
        Abdominal Pain. BMJ **2**: 73-75, 1975.

C

A simplified version of a system for computer-aided diagnosis of acute abdominal pain has been tested by new personnel unfamiliar with the previous system. The findings validate further the concept of the computer as a potential valuable diagnostic aid, but indicate that a training period and computer feedback are important factors in its use.

[75]   De Dombal FT, Horrocks JC: Computer-aided Diagnosis:
        Conclusions from an overall Experience Involving 4469 patients.
        MEDINFO 74: 581-585, Almqvist & Wiksell, 1974.

C

A report from a computer-aided diagnostic system developed in Leeds uses a Bayesian probabilistic analysis in an adaptable format with conditional probabilities derived from prior, large-scale, clinical studies. Comparative prospective studies have been carried out. The cost effectiveness of the system has been assessed according to some of the available parameters. It is likely it economises in the use of hospital beds and may prevent unnecessary operations.

[76]   De Dombal FT et al: Human and Computer Aided Diagnosis of
        Abdominal Pain: Further report with emphasis on Performance of
        Clinicians. BMJ **1**: 376-380, 1974.

C

A trial which evaluates the effectiveness of the different diagnostic processes was conducted. It is suggested that, while computer-aided diagnosis is a valuable, direct adjunct to the clinician dealing with the "acute abdomen", he may also benefit in the short term from the constant feedback he receives and from the disciplines and constraints involved in communicating with the computer.

[77]   De Dombal FT et al: Simulation of Clinical Diagnosis: A comparative
        study. BMJ **2**: 575-577, 1971.

C

A comparison of three different modes of diagnosis simulation, one being computer based. The need for an acceptable simulation remains. Future simulations should be flexible, economical, and acceptably realistic - and this implies (in the study) a two-way use of speech. Such a system is currently being built and tested.

[78]   De Dombal FT et al: Computer aided Diagnosis of Acute Abdominal
        Pain. BMJ **2**: 9-13, 1972.

C

This paper reports a controlled prospective unselected real-time
comparison of human and computer-aided diagnosis. The report suggests that the provision of such a system to aid the clinician is both feasible in a real-time clinical setting and likely to be of practical value, albeit in a small percentage of cases.

[79]   De Dombal FT: Computer-Assisted Diagnosis of Abdominal Pain using
        "Estimates" Provided by Clinicians. BMJ **4**: 350-354, 1972.

244

C

A report of a comparison between two modes of computer aided diagnosis in a real-time trial. Using real life data the computer was significantly more effective than the unaided physician. It seems that future systems for computer aided diagnosis should employ data from real-life and not clinicians' estimates, and also that physicians themselves cannot analyse cases in a probabilistic fashion since often they have little idea of what the two probabilities are.

[80]   Degoulet P et al: Patient Compliance in hypertension care: the critical role of the computer. MIE 82: 288-295, Springer-Verlag, 1982.

F

The role of the computer in improving patient compliance with the medical treatment of arterial hypertension is analysed in the light of the experience obtained with the computerised ARTEMIS system. The efforts required include organisational, educational, and therapeutic measures, as well as perseverance in identifying the factors associated with poor compliance.

[81]   De Moel J: General Practitioners' Information Systems: An Information System for Practice, Management, Research. MEDINFO 83, 1177-1180, North-Holland, 1983.

E/F

A description of a system applicable for practice management and medical registration, as well as for research in the field of epidemiology and health service research. The systems specifications are presented. Additionally problems that arise from the combined approach are discussed.

[82]   De Moel J: General Practitioners Information System. MIE 82, 306-308, Springer-Verlag, 1982.

E

A look at a GP information system employed in the Netherlands which is intended to serve two major objectives viz to support the provision of information within general practices, and further to provide an instrument to facilitate health service research.

[83]   Dezelic GJ et al: Computer Assisted Instruction in Continuing Education for Primary Health Care: Project Concepts and Development. MEDINFO 89, 1078-1082, North-Holland, 1989.

I

This new system of continuing education in primary health care is based on the use of electronic (video and computer) technology. The computer part of the system is oriented to the use of CAI methods. The concepts of CAI in continuing education for PHC are presented, and the main results achieved, as well as the perspectives of future development, are discussed.

[84]   Dezelic GJ et al: Development of health information systems for health centres delivering primary care in distributed environment. MIE 87, 203-208, EDI Press, Rome, 1987.

G

The basic problems in developing this kind of system are explored and the design principles of such a system proposed with consideration of the economic constraints of the primary health care environment.

[85]   Dezelic GJ et al: Development of a health data base for analysing the relation between environmental health and medical data with a micro computer. MIE 88: 185-189, Springer-Verlag, 1988.

G

This database is planned to be part of a distributed information system in primary health care. Discussed are ecological analyses performed from mortality and morbidity data, and from information collected in daily primary health care work. The advantages of the last approach are pointed out.

[86]   DHSS: Survey of computerised general practices. NHS Info Tech Branch, 1987.

E

This report gives the results of a questionnaire survey to discover why practices had bought systems, what tasks they performed, and what further development they desired.

[87]   DHSS: Joint Policy Computer Group. Micros in Practice: report of an appraisal of GP Micro Computer Systems. DHSS London HMSO, 1986.

E

This study aims to provide doctors with objective information concerning currently available micro computer systems including technical performance and of the use of systems by GPs and their staff. The report aims to increase awareness of microcomputer applications and enable doctors to make more informed decisions about the purchase of such computer systems.

[88]   DHSS: Final Report. Project Evaluation Group. General Practice Computing - evaluation of the "Micro for GPs" scheme, London: HMSO, 1985.

E

A report of the scheme designed to promote awareness of IT in general medical practice which covers a number of important topics including implementation of systems, reliability, registration of patients, recall, prescribing, as well as patient attitudes to computers and factors affecting their success.

[89]   Difford F: Future trends in general practice computing. JRCGP **37**: 434-435, 1987.

I

A look at what wider developments practices would like to see in future including electronic mail, data links to hospitals and FPC, and computer readable medical cards.

[90]   Difford F: A computerised audit of a screening programme to establish rubella immunity. JRCGP **36**: 371 - 372, 1986.

F

This paper reports the use of a practice computer to help establish rubella immunity in all women that are likely to bear children. Results of successive audits show consistent increases in the numbers of women with established rubella immunity.

[91]   Difford F: Reducing Prescription Costs through computer controlled repeat prescribing. JRCGP **34**: 658-660, 1984.

C

A small reduction in prescribing costs are reported from a practice that has been using a computerised repeat-prescribing system for three years. The possible reasons for this are discussed.

[92]   Difford F et al: Continuous opportunistic and systematic screening for hypertension with computer help: analysis of non-responders. BMJ **294**: 1130-1132, 1987.

F

For two years a computer was used to identify patients, to prompt for opportunistic screening, and to call for systematic screening. With the help of a micro-computer it is practicable to sustain a continuous screening rate of between 90% and 95%.

[93]   Difford F: Mapping practice population and morbidity with a computer. BMJ **291**: 1017-1020, 1985.

E

A method of dividing a map of the practice area into a grid based on postcodes is described. The distribution of the practice population may thus be shown graphically and trends observed. The geographical incidence of, and prevalence of, morbidity may also be charted and variations of statistical significance determined. This is a practical tool that will have greater potential as information technology in general practice develops.

[94]   Difford F et al: Maintaining the accuracy of a computer practice register: household index. BMJ **290**: 519-521, 1985.

D/E/F

In a practice of 9726 patients, a computer is used for recall, screening, morbidity data, audit and repeat-prescribing. The computing techniques used to achieve accuracy in maintaining the register are described. After one year the computer register was validated by using the computer to randomly select 200 patients' records that had not been updated recently. Results indicated that it is feasible and valuable to have a household index.

[95]   Difford F: Computer controlled repeat prescribing used to analyse drug management. BMJ **289**: 593-595, 1984.

D

A method is described in which, for given diagnoses, the computer can identify the appropriate drugs and add them together in a systematic way to produce detailed printouts of the drug management in the practice. A technique by which the computer user can analyse them further on a pharmacological basis is shown.

[96]   Dinklo JA: Confidentiality of Medical Data in the Usage of Data Banks. MEDINFO 74: 181-187, Almqvist & Wiksell, 1974.

B

Consideration of the protection of patients' medical data and methods to improve security of that data when stored by electronic means.

[97]   Dinwoodie HP, Howell RW: Automatic disease coding; the 'fruit machine' method in general practice. Br J Prev Soc Med **27** (1), 59 - 62, 1973.

E/F

The problems and benefits of automatic coding of general practice data are similar to those of hospital discharge-summaries and are centred on machine costs versus the undoubted efficiency and speed of machine coding. Nevertheless it seems desirable to illustrate the principle of automatic disease coding as applied to general practice.

[98]   Dodge JR: Auditing a computer based immunisation programme. Current Perspectives in HC: 41-52, BJHC, 1985.

F

The potential of a computer-based child health programme has been realised for providing service management information.   From this considerable improvements in the immunisation program are encouraging further expansion of the monitoring role. The methodology is described and illustrated.

[99]   Donald JB: Prescribing costs when computers are used to issue all prescriptions. BMJ **299**: 28-30, 1989.

D

The aim of this study was to see whether the user of computers to issue prescriptions in conjunction with a computerised, customised drug formulary affects prescribing costs. The report concludes that prescribing costs were reduced when a computer was used to issue all prescriptions in conjunction with a personal, computerised formulary.

[100]   Donald JB: On line prescribing by computer. BMJ **292**: 937-939, 1986.

D

A computer is used to produce all prescriptions for patients seen in the consulting room in this practice. The method saves time, improves safety, decreases prescribing costs, and provides an instant audit of all important prescribing parameters. Treatment is rationalised and patients are given an improved service. The savings in costs are not likely to be substantial; however, when all prescribing is done by computer from a limited drug formulary, these savings may be appreciable.

[101]   Doroba A, Leligdowicz A: Two year experience in problem oriented records of primary health care. MEDINFO 77: 479-480, North-Holland, 1977.

A

The results of a pilot project dealing with problem oriented medical records are presented and discussed. This project took place in seven primary health regions over a 2 year period.

[102]   Dove G et al: General-practice history taking by computer: A "psychotropic" effect. MIE 79: 253-260, Springer-Verlag, 1979.

C

This paper is the report of an experiment in the use of a computer for interviewing patients in general practice, in order to obtain their social and medical history, and the conclusions formed as a result. Research shows that comprehensive history taking interviews by computers can have beneficial effects which were not expected from such an impersonal form of communication.

[103]   Dove GA et al: The therapeutic effect of taking a patient's history by computer. JRCGP **27**: 477-481, 1977.

C

A report which suggests that the benefits of a computer history taking system could be extended to all classes of society.

[104]   Dove G, Norris P: Reflections on an interactive computerised history taking system in a general medical practice. MIE 82: 280-284, Springer-Verlag, 1982.

C

An interactive microcomputer-based questionnaire has been devised, using simple friendly language, to interview patients in a general profile. The social history obtained from the programme was made available to the doctor before his subsequent consultation with the patient. The paper explores the nature of the patient's experience with the computer and the implications for future medical practice.

[105]   Downs SM et al: Automated Summarisation of On-Line Medical Records. MEDINFO 86: 800-804, North-Holland , 1986.

A

Such summaries represent an important advance and provide a useful addition to medical records for clinical decision making, real-time patient monitoring, or surveillance of quality of care. This paper describes a design for automated summarisation in time-oriented medical records of systemic lupus erythematosus patients. The interface allows convenient, interactive exploration of the data, user modelling, and the ability of the system to explain its reasoning.

[106]   Ducrot H: Conditions of Use of Drug Information Systems designed for physicians or pharmacists. MEDINFO 83: 134, North-Holland, 1983.

D

Computerised systems, for the mentioned users, must be designed so that they can be easily integrated into daily practice. They will always result in a compromise between complete systems, unusable because of their complexity, and less elaborate systems which are easier to understand. This paper addresses key questions involved with such systems.

[107]   Duisterhout JS, Branger PJ: Communication in Primary Care Systems. MEDINFO 89: 700-703, North-Holland , 1989.

G

Communication plays an important role in health care. The use of electronic information reduces loss of information in the communication process due to transcription errors. It allows for faster communication, and makes information available at multiple places at the same time. Standard message formats, message types, and data items allow for exchange of information between different health care information systems. The paper looks at the areas of communication and the COPA Project.

[108]   Dvergsdal P: Interactive patient record. MIE 85: 404-409, Springer-Verlag , 1985.

A

This paper describes a computerised medical record system. Each patient's record is integrated using a menu of about 500 standard medical texts. With these it is possible to achieve semi-automatic writing of medical records and communications to be sent or handed to patients.

[109]   Ellis D: Medical Computing and Applications. Ellis Harwood, 1987.

C/E/I

A detailed account of the growth of medical computing. Coverage includes diagnosis and patient management, and the role of computers in specialised areas of medicine. Chapter 4 is a critique of progress in GP computing.

[110]   Ewins DL et al: Computerised updating of clinical summaries: new opportunities for clinical practice and research. BMJ **297**: 1504-1506, 1988.

A

Even completely new computerised summaries are quicker to produce than conventional summaries and computerised summaries are designed to be scanned rapidly for relevant information. They can also be used for collecting data automatically for research, clinical audit, and resource management.

[111]   Farmer RD, Grosc KW: An automated records system for general practice. Br J Prev Soc Med **26** (3): 148 - 152, 1972.

A An automated records system is described which is designed to limit the Health Service usage by a population registered with a group of general practitioners, and to assist in the administration of the services they are providing.

[112]   Fell PJ, Skees WD: The Doctor's Computer Handbook. Lifetime Learning Publications, 1984.

E

The book is written for the physician wishing to computerise a medical practice and best suits those looking beyond off-the-shelf products to a system adapted to their particular practice needs. The book provides the information essential to making such decisions. Its goal is to help readers understand how a vendor's system can be customised to serve the doctors specific needs from an administrative and clinical standpoint.

[113]   Fisher RH: The role of FPS computing with regard to the problems of patient care computing as a whole. Current Perspectives in HC: 221-229, BJHC,1984.

G

This presents a forecast of the overall health care computing scenario; written at a time when major changes were expected.

[114]   Fitter MJ et al: A human factors evaluation of the IBM Sheffield Primary Care System. INTERACT **84**: 675 - 681, 1984.

E The paper reports on an evaluation focusing on the 'human factors' aspects of designing and implementing a complex and comprehensive information system in an unfamiliar and relatively unstructured environment. Certain specific problems resulting from the design of the interface arose. However, they were minor and in this respect the system was well liked. The most significant issues arose from the organisational impact and the mismatch between the systems and the user organisation.

[115]   Fitter MJ, Garber R: (Repeat Prescription) - Is It Worth It? Practice Computing **3**(3): 19-25, June 1984.

D

Repeat prescriptions are seen as ideal candidates for computerisation, but the conclusions of one large practice indicate that the task is not trouble-free.

[116]   Fitter MJ: Making GP computers effective. BJHC: November 1986.

E

General practitioners should only compute when they are already well organised and are sure of their reasons for doing so. The summarised findings of a DHSS report are presented.

[117]   Fitter MJ, Garber et al. (eds.): A Prescription for Change. - A report on the longer term use and development of computers in General Practice. London: HMSO, 1986.

E

A study which compares practices with computers installed and practices without computers. The aim is to assess the impact of computers on the practices, their ability to support improved health care delivery, and factors that support or impede progress.

[118]   Fitter MJ et al: Computers and audit. JRCGP **35**: 522-524, 1985.

H

The paper describes how a computerised information system, installed in a large group practice, was used for the systematic audit of clinical activities and also demonstrates how it acted as a catalyst for the review and changes of administrative and management procedures.

[119]   Fox J, Alvey P: Computer assisted medical decision making. BMJ **287**: 742-745, 1983.

C

The main problem here lies in the development of a reliable and acceptable method of reasoning about stored facts. Initially statistical analysis was used, and such systems have been extensively developed and tested. More recently attention has shifted to the use of logic for manipulating facts expressed in qualitative terms. These knowledge-based techniques are still in their infancy but already show signs of exciting potential.

[120] Furukawa T: Theory in Computer-Aided Diagnosis. MEDINFO 80: 750-753, North-Holland , 1980.

C

An introductory set of remarks on the subject looking at the advances and concepts of application of computer-aided diagnosis.

[121] Gallen D: Don't buy a computer unless you research it. Financial Pulse, May 23 1989: 22-25.

E

A personal view from a six-handed practice, on how they computerised. This, the first article in a series, describes how the practice chose a system which they thought was value for money.

[122] Gallen D: Practice progress: next create your own database. Financial Pulse, June 6, 1989: 35-36.

E

The second article in the series explains that, having decided which computer system to go for, the next decision facing members of the practice team was how to create the patient database.

[123] Gallen D: Installation day ... the trials of the first weeks. Financial Pulse, June 20, 1989: 41.

E

In this article, the third in the series following the computerisation of a practice, it is explained how the computer system was installed and outlines the practice's enterprising training strategy.

[124] Gallen D: Theory to practice with our computers. Financial Pulse, August 15, 1989: 35.

E

This article, continuing a series following the computerisation of a practice, looks at how the computer system is helping with organisation several months after installation.

[125] GMSC: Computers in General Practice. BMJ **280**: 662-663, 1980.

E

Outlines what the GMS Committee expects from the study commissioned, to be undertaken by Scicon - a firm of computer consultants.

[126] GMSC: GMSC advises on computer contracts. BMJ **295**: 281, 1987.

E

The GMSC has advised general practitioners of the steps they should take before entering into contracts with AAH-Meditel and VAMP, which have offered to provide computers free of charge.

[127] GMSC/RCGP Joint Computing Policy Group: 1982 Report. BMJ **286**: 660-661, 1983.

I

This report describes the progress in matters initiated in 1981 and the Committee's recommendations and subsequent action in 1982.

[128] GMSC/RCGP Joint Policy Computing Group: 1983 Report. BMJ **289**: 1242, 1984.

I

The third year of the group's activity has been accompanied by a rapidly increasing interest in computers by general practitioners.

[129] GMSC/RCGP Joint Computing Policy Group: BMJ **290**: 1252-1253, 1985.

D

A number of essential and recommended standards for the issue of computerised prescriptions are described.

[130] GMSC/RCGP Joint Computing Policy Group: Standards for computer issued prescriptions. Research and Development in Primary Care computing. JRCGP **32**: 88-92, 1982.

I

The policy groups view about needs for research and development in primary health care. The paper excludes any suggestions about mechanisms through which the research may be conducted. It is intended as a guide to those who may be contemplating research and development in this field, and to bodies who may be requested to fund such activities.

[131] GMSC/RCGP Joint Policy Computing Group: General Practice Report for 1981. JRCGP **32**: 197-198, 1982.

I

A report on the first meeting of the group.

[132] Grace JF: A Computer in your practice: indispensable tool or troublesome toy? BMJ **285**: 1169-1171, 1982.

E

This is an enlightenment on the advantages, disadvantages, pleasures, curses, savings, and expense of installing a packaged computer system into a busy general practice. It gives a chronological account of the problems in one practice and the position of the computer in that practice one year after installation.

[133] Grant D: Record linkage in general practice: the computers in medical records. Practitioner **204**: 444 - 5, 1970.

A This paper consists of several articles looking at the problem of scattered medical records and the need to link all these records together by the use of data banks and incorporate processing. There are also sections looking at related issues such as confidentiality.

[134] Grene JD, Henderson JM: Automated recall in general practice. JRCGP **21**: 352-355, 1971.

E/F

Automatic recall, initially by a punch card index and later by computer, has been used to follow-up patients in a group practice. A hospital computer scheme was modified for this purpose and found to be too sophisticated for the small area of a practice.

[135]   Griesser G (ed.) et al: Data Protection in health information systems. North Holland, 1980.

B

The text starts with a description and explanation of the key elements of the problem. Subsequent chapters address issues relating to certain groups of people, i.e. professionals, involved in the usage of data, and those responsible for enforcing standards. The existing laws on data protection are explained as well as suggestions for selection of data protection measures with regard to economic aspects.

[136]   Griesser G: Data Protection in Health Information Systems, MEDINFO 83: 950-953, North-Holland , 1983.

B

The requirement of safeguarding the patients' claim to secrecy of all data entrusted to a physician and his assistants is the basis of a trusted patient-physician relationship. To meet this requirement and to ensure data and programs are not lost or altered inadvertently, an exact risk analysis of computer-based information systems is indispensable for the planning and design of a comprehensive system of data protection measures consisting of hardware precautions, software techniques, and organisational arrangements. This paper discusses the problem.

[137]   Griesser G, Kenny D: Constructing guidelines for data protection in health information systems. MIE 79: 80-82, Springer-Verlag , 1979.

B

It is in the interests of patients, doctors, computer specialists and administrators, that the whole matter concerning data protection is examined in the correct context and robust solutions devised to meet the oncoming problems. It is particularly important at this juncture to learn how to map out the difficult ground which lies between government action and the local technical precautions devised by the DP manager.

[138]   Gruer KT: Livingstone New Town - Using a computer for general practice records. JRCGP **22**: 100-107, 1972.

A/G

This system is part of an experimental project which aims to create an area health service based on health centres and supported by a community oriented hospital. A new role has been devised for the GP in which he has both a community and hospital commitment. This paper is a look at the computer concept and uses.

[139]   Gruer KT, Heasman MA: Livingstone New Town - Use of computer in general practice medical records. BMJ **2**: 289-291, 1970.

A

The GPs involved work from a health centre and each also holds a hospital appointment. The most effective assistance provided so far by the computer is in the preventative field

254

of the practitioners work. Equally important potential use is in the processing of data in such a way as to allow the doctor to assess his method of work and to provide information of statistical and epidemiological value.

[140]   Gunner C: The implications of smart card technology. Current Perspectives in HC: 236-240, BJHC, 1988.

A/I

More emphasis is being placed on the improvement of communications between patient data and practitioners and the health service. The smart card offers a new level of communication that is already being applied in continental Europe and the US. During 1988 trials in this technology will start in the UK. This paper introduces what a smart card is and addresses how it is being used today and what is the likely future direction.

[141]   Hall J: A future strategy for FPS Computing. Current Perspectives in HC: 224-234, BJHC, 1985.

G

The DHSS published a study by Arthur Anderson & Co. concerning FPS administration and the use of computers in July 1984. This paper describes the major conclusions of the study and highlights the potential implications for health authorities.

[142]   Handby JG: Computerising Family Practitioner Services. MIE 85: 373-379, Springer-Verlag , 1985.

G

The paper outlines the proposals and plans of the DHSS/NHS to go ahead with the proposals contained in the report by Arthur Anderson & Co. which advises on the future development of computer systems within the FPS.

[143]   Handby JG: Harnessing Technology to health care - the challenge for the future. MIE 84: 616-621, Springer-Verlag , 1984.

I

With specific reference to the Health Service in England, the paper presents a view of where the use of technology stands at present, and what the future prospects are, and what is needed to realise them.

[144]   Hannaford PC, Hawkins TJ: Computer Support for Patient Management. Current Perspectives in HC: 85-89, BJHC, 1988.

H

One popular task for computers is to review a series of pre-ordained tasks, to identify discrepancies, and to bring these to the notice of a controller. A protocol for disease management can be thought of as such a pre-ordained task. The advantages of computers are discussed and illustrated.

[145]   Hannay DR, Mitchell S: Storing Summary Patient Data as a Microcomputer File. JRCGP **35**: 525-526, 1985.

A

A summary of the evaluation of the time taken to summarise 1000 patient records and store this data as a hard disc file on a microcomputer in a health centre with about 7300 patients.

[146]   Harding N: Data Protection in Medicine. TL Visuals, 1986.

B

A national meeting was held at John Radcliffe Hospital, Oxford in February 1986. This book covers the proceedings which relate to data protection in the medical profession as a whole. However specific chapters are dedicated to General Practice and Primary Health Care and the author discusses the implications of the Data Protection Act.

[147]   Hardy RH: Can I Computerise you now, Sir? JRCGP **15**: 233-237, 1968.

E

A point of view from the author.

[148]   Hargrave L et al: Computerised Family Practitioner Committee Records - a data base for general practice. JRCGP **38**: 22-23, 1988.

E/G

In PHC preventative medicine is becoming increasingly important, and GPs need up-to-date accurate information about their practice population. The paper examines a study carried out in Northumberland to establish the type of information which could be of interest to GPs and how it could be produced.

[149]   Hayes G: Data and Doctors. BJHC February 1989.

B

A look at the areas of the Data Protection Act 1984 that concern general practitioners.

[150]   Hedley A et al: Computer-assisted Follow Up Register for the NE of Scotland. BMJ **1**: 556-558, 1970.

F

An automated follow up register for the detection of iatrogenic thyroid disease has been established as a joint venture between GPs and a thyroid clinic. Patients are followed up and the system is designed to process, screen, and store clinical and biochemical follow-up data and report results to patients, GPs, and the hospital records department.

[151]   Henderson J: Instant age-sex register. BMJ **288**: 1967-1968, 1984.

A

An age-sex register for use in general practice was obtained directly from the Family Practitioner Committee Computer by direct transfer of data to a microcomputer.

[152]   Herd A: Multi - user systems: Panacea or pain in the neck? Practice Computing. 7 - 9, November 1989.

E A member of the primary health care specialist group of the BCS shares his misgivings about too early acceptance of multi-user systems in general practice.

[153]   Grene JD: Computer Compatible records in general practice. JRCGP **19**: 29-33, 1970.

A

By finding out the snags of recording information in computer compatible form, the author tries to answer the question "how can the general practitioner modify his methods of record keeping to ensure that the maximum help can be obtained from the computer".

[154]   Herzmark G et al: Consultation use of a computer by general practitioners. JRCGP **34**: 649-654, 1984.

C

This study focuses primarily on the experiences of doctors in their efforts to communicate with patients and computers concurrently, and the differences a computer makes in the consultation.

[155]   Heyrman J: Computerisation of the medical record of the general practitioner: systematic registration at each patient-gp contact.

MIE 78: 101-108, Springer-Verlag , 1978.

A

A two year investigation about the possibilities of centralising all medical data around the patient, links up with the fact that one may expect that the use of a similar registration system by the GP and the specialist can prevent somewhat the problems of the information gap, and double-use, or even loss of, medical data.

[156]   Hodgkin P: Reading the printout on the wall: decision making in general practice. BMJ **288**: 198-199, 1984.

C

A report from a conference which brought together ordinary GPs, those who are designing medical software, psychologists, and social scientists who have been looking at how doctors make decisions. The conference concentrated on the application of computers as decision aids.

[157]   Hogkinson M: Practice Computers. JRCGP **36**: 535, 1986.

E

The RCGP's information technology manager explains how the College can help with crucial advice on the important purchase of a business computer for general practice.

[158]   Horn W: ESDAT - Decision Support for primary medical care. MEDINFO 83: 484-487, North-Holland , 1983.

C

ESDAT is a decision support system designed for application in primary medical care. It represents medical knowledge in a semantic net. The symbolic reasoning process of the system activates disease hypotheses from this net. These hypotheses are candidates for confirmation or rejection. Major emphasis is put on focusing mechanisms.

[159]   Horrocks JC, De Dombal FT: Diagnosis of Dyspepsia from Data collected by a Physician's assistant. BMJ **3**: 421-423, 1975.

C

This paper presents a study of the diagnosis of dyspepsia in 154 patients based on data collected at their initial outpatient attendance by an interview with a non-medically qualified assistant. The results were positive and conclude (1) the data recorded was diagnostically valuable, (2) when necessary the information collection can be delegated to a non-medically qualified person; but (3) this interview should augment and not replace the traditional interview by the physician.

[160]   Horrocks JC et al: Computer Aided Diagnosis: Description of an Adaptable System and Operational Experience with 2,034 cases. BMJ **2**: 5-9, 1972.

C

This paper describes a system of computer-aided diagnosis using a computer linked to a terminal in a busy clinical department. Data from a series of patients was recorded, coded, and entered into the computer, which then performed some analysis and displayed diagnostic probabilities in an adaptable format. Experience in this setting suggests that computer diagnosis may be a valuable aid to the clinician.

[161]   Houghton KA: Integrated data and opportunities for improving care. Current Perspectives in HC: 129-132, BJHC,1987.

G

This paper considers the merits of using aggregated data (in FPS and community health service systems), for planning the provision of services and monitoring how services are delivered to patients.

[162]   Howarth FP: Micros for GPs. BMJ **292**: 307-308, 1986.

E

A brief summary of the successes and shortcomings of the micros for GPs scheme, nearly four years old.

[163]   Howkins TJ, Kay CR: A computer-based appointment system for general practice. MEDINFO 89: 991-994, North-Holland , 1989.

E/H

Most general practices organise their clinician-patient contact by some form of appointment system. The use of computers has focused on computer based appointment systems. In response to this, a research program was started to build a general practice computer system based on an appointments system. This was completed in 1986 and this paper looks at the provisions of the system, the experience of using it over the last two years, its statistical potential and the applicability of this system's philosophy in primary and secondary health care.

[164]   Hunday DS: Applications of personal computers in general practice. MIE 84: 565-566, Springer-Verlag , 1984.

E

A short paper which points out some of the common applications that personal computers can attend to in a practice.

[165]   Ingram JA, Asbury AJ: Patient Administration - I/II. BMJ **287**: 600-603/667-670, 1983.

H

A detailed look at various implementations of patient administration systems, their development, and links to other systems and the advantages achievable.

[166]   Irwin WG et al: Effect on prescribing of the limited list in a computerised group practice. BMJ **293**: 857-859, 1986.

D

The prescription of drugs in the therapeutic classes that are affected by the government's limited list was investigated in a computerised practice of just over 3000 patients. The results are contained within the report.

[167]   Janecki J, Kokott H: Experiments with medical diagnostic systems. MIE 78: 29-36, Springer-Verlag , 1978.

C

This paper's aim was to check what influence changes of certain parameters has on the efficiency of a simple system of differential diagnosis.

[168]   Jarman B: Giving advice about welfare benefits in general practice. BMJ **290:** 522-524, 1985.

E

General Practitioners and community nurses are exceptionally well placed to detect those suffering genuine financial hardship but they are not well equipped to give advice about the complex system of state social security benefits. A method of providing such advice in a health centre with the help of a computer is described.

[169]   Jelovsek FR: Doctor's Office Computer Prep Kit. Springer-Verlag, New York, 1985.

E

This provides clinical advice to physicians who are planning to purchase an office practice computer and includes an analysis of the features available in office practice billing systems. It also emphasises the nature of the billing process and alternatives. It is a primer about the ins and outs of billing for any physician about to set up in practice.

[170]   Johnson RA: Computer analysis of the complete medical record including symptoms and treatment. JRCGP **22**: 655-660, 1972.

A/I

Problems of definition of the area of work and the establishment of a medical data bank are the main stumbling blocks of medical computing. A method of improving medical computing is suggested.

[171]   Kay S, Davis R: How one GP computer system survived. Current Perspectives in HC: 148-154, BJHC, 1987.

E

Describes how the University of Wales embarked on a new course by establishing a computer-based information system for general practice in 1968 and describes the trials and developments since.

[172]   Kayll J: The computer key to information in general practice. Current Perspectives in HC: 37-48, BJHC, 1986.

E

This is a report on the long term benefits that have accrued to a general practice over a period of three years use of a mature, second generation computer: VAMP Health's Integrated General Practice (VAMP IGP).

[173]   Keating J: GP acceptance of computer-generated hospital discharge letters. Current Perspectives in HC: 32, BJHC, 1989.

E/G

Computer generated discharge letters are an acceptable alternative to conventional hospital discharge letters in patients discharged from general surgical wards. They have the advantage of saving time by avoiding duplication of information if this has already been collected for the purpose of computerised audit.

[174]   Klaring WJ: CAPOS - Computer-aided physicians' office system. MIE 82: 285-287, Springer-Verlag , 1982.

H

It is possible to manage the numerous tasks of a surgery rationally with the help of computerised organisation systems that are carefully planned and optimally adapted to the individual demands, and in such a way as to save time and money. Philosophies, strategies and possible uses of CAPOS are discussed.

[175]   Kopjar B et al: A micro-computer based problem-oriented medical record system for PHC. MIE 88: 207-210, Springer-Verlag , 1988.

A

It has been recognised that existing manual health information systems cannot satisfy modern information requirements in PHC and that the remedy should be in an information system based on computer technology. The aim of this work is to develop a model for a medical record suitable for computerised health information systems in PHC.

[176]   Kumpel Z: Referral letters - the enclosure of the general practitioner's computerised record. JRCGP **28**: 163-167, 1978.

A

The computerisation of general practice records in group practices often makes it possible for a print-out of the record to be sent to hospital specialists on referral. The value of this has been assessed by consultants. GPs and consultants do not agree on the content of the ideal referral letter; the addition of a computer print-out would aid about a third of consultants.

[177]   Kurashina S: Comparative Study of Computer-Aided Clinical Decision Making Systems. MEDINFO 80: 825-829, North-Holland , 1980.

C

This paper reports a comparative and experimental field study on the usefulness of some of these systems. Although such systems differ among each other in their problem field, design considerations, and developmental stages, the study gives several important insights into such systems and lists design considerations useful for future development of such systems.

260

[178]   Law J: Sell your practice data at profit. Medeconomics: June 1987.

A

Computerised patient records can be worth a lot of money to GPs as well as providing an invaluable basis for improving medical care.

[179]   Law J: Manage to get the most from a computer. Medeconomics:
         December 1986.

H

Effective computing is about good management. A practice manager with an organised approach showed nine GPs how they could make their computers work for their individual needs.

[180]   Lawrence M: A computer generated patient carried health check
         card. JRCGP **36:** 458-460, 1986.

A

A system has been developed so that a patient's important medical information can be printed out and be given to the patient in the form of a health check card. One aim was to encourage patients to take more responsibility for their own preventative care.

[181]   Leaper DJ et al: Clinical Diagnostic Process: An Analysis. BMJ **3:**
         569-574, 1973.

C

An analysis of observations made during diagnosis of 1307 patients by 28 clinicians. Interviews were conducted in a variety of different ways. The study concludes that automated diagnostic systems must be flexible to accommodate the wishes of a variety of clinicians.

[182]   Lewis A: Coming to terms with computers. Practitioner **231:** 1275 -
         78,   October 8th 1987.

E Computerisation offers many advances in ease and quality of patients care. Computerisation results in improved recall systems and in better self and practice audit. Easier transfer of data between practice and FPC will result from the computerisation of FPC data. Difficulties with computerisation come partly from resistance to change, but these can largely be overcome by the successful management of change.

[183]   Limik B, Srdanovic V: An expert consultation system to aid clinical
         diagnoses. MIE 85: 138-142, Springer-Verlag , 1985.

C

An expert consultation system to support clinical decision making has been developed. Medical expert knowledge and data from clinical practice are combined to comprise the knowledge base of the system. The system has originally been designated to deal with problems in rheumatology, and it has been tested successfully.

[184]   Linnarsson R: Development and evaluation of a complete
         computer-based problem-oriented medical record system for primary
         care. MIE 87: 209-214, EDI Press, Rome, 1987.

A

Computerised information systems in medical care have usually concentrated on administrative functions. The consequence of this is that systems for medical information processing are rare and it is difficult to expand an administrative system to include clinical functions. The basic approach in the project described here is to give priority to the medical record and to let the administrative routines be gradually automated later.

[185]   Lipman EO, Preece JF: A pilot on-line data system for general practitioners. Comput Biomed Res **4** (4): 309 - 406, 1971.

A

A description of the design and implementation of the system which is designed to enable general practitioners to create, access, and maintain centrally stored clinical records via remote terminal devices.

[186]   Lloyd SC: Computer-generated progress notes in an automated POMR. J Med. Syst. **8**(1-2): 35-42, 1984.

A

This extended version of the Weed system is regularly used by primary care physicians. The method is an extension of the POMR system of keeping medical records.

[187]   Lockley WJ: Mediscreen - a database for general practice. Current Perspectives in HC: 31-36, BJHC, 1986.

E

GPs are expected to absorb new information all the time from all spheres of medicine as well as a knowledge of other related disciplines - the volume of new data is incredibly vast. However if a speedily updated, readily accessible, mechanical database were available, tailored for GPs use, then GPs would become aware that they could treat with confidence a much wider range of problems. This paper describes MEDISCREEN, which sets out to be that data base.

[188]   Lucas R et al: Computer Interrogation of Patients. BMJ **2**: 623-625, 1976.

C

A system of routine interrogation of patients using a computer has been developed. It consists of a visual display unit and a specially designed response keyboard. The system was evaluated using the criteria of accuracy in eliciting symptoms, acceptability to the patient, and cost. While doctors will always take the ultimate management decisions, it seems that machines can be programmed to undertake interrogation of patients, elicit evidence accurately and acceptably as effectively as doctors.

[189]   MacQueen D: Implications of primary health data capture. Current Perspectives in HC: 90-94, BJHC, 1988.

C

Clinical decision making can be categorised in terms of costs and benefits primarily concerned with quality of patient care and how best to deal with each prognosis. They are also concerned with efficiency in the use of resources and equity in the process of selection. Clearly the availability of reliable data is a fundamental pre-requisite for the controlled management of vital resources. The question of how to translate data into effective information for health care management is quite another matter.

[190]   Madeley RJ, Metcalfe DW: Doctors' attitudes to information systems - a survey of Derbyshire's general practitioners. JRCGP **28**: 654-658, 1978.

E

This paper deals with,in particular, GPs attitudes to IS and the factors which affect them. The results show that there is much more interest in continuous data collection from primary care than is often supposed. This is particularly so among young GPs. The survey describes the possible interest in information recording amongst a typical population of GPs.

[191]   Malcolm A, Poyser J: Computers and the General Practitioner (Proceedings of the GP-Info Symposium). London Pergamon Press, 1980.

E

In 1980 the RCGP held a symposium (GP-INF0-80) to enable those pioneering the field of medical computing to promote and discuss their work with potential users. This book contains edited versions of papers concerning the present and potential role of computers in general practice. The book covers most of the contemporary issues related to computers and primary health care.

[192]   Malmberg BG: A complete medical record system and its Data Dictionary, used by General Practitioners and district nurses, working in a district health centre. MIE 87: 215-224, EDI Press, Rome, 1987.

A

A background and discussion of the goals, achievements and advantages of a system actually in use and the procedures it uses.

[193]   Mann N: Smart Cards in Health Care: A solution in search of a problem. MEDINFO 89: 1151-1155, North-Holland , 1989.

A/I

Smart cards have sparked considerable interest in the past four years in the health care industry. They face few technical problems but incentives for their use are weak or lacking. As a result their use is limited to specific functions extending current products such as claims processing. The paper looks at the potential use of this technology and at some barriers to its use.

[194]   Marcus A: A plan for information in the National Health Service. Lancet **2**: 1242-1243, 1988.

E

A look at general practices and their suitability for computerisation, and the influence computerisation could have on the services of general practices.

[195]   Masterman L: FPS Computerisation - the past, the present and the future. Current Perspectives in HC: 35, BJHC, 1989.

G

This paper outlines the way computing in the FPS has developed, from hesitant beginnings, to its present position of reasonable strength; and how it is poised to influence the future to benefit all associated with the FPS - practitioners, patients and administrators.

[196]   McAlister NH et al: Randomised Controlled trial of computer assisted management of hypertension in primary care. BMJ **293**: 670-674, 1986.

F/H

The hypothesis that general practitioners would obtain better outcomes for patients with hypertension using a computer than doctors not using a computer was tested. The results are in this report.

[197]   McCurry MG: Large scale implementation of FPS computer systems in England and Wales. MIE 88: 473-477, Springer-Verlag , 1988.

G/I

In 1983 a report recommended the computerising of the family practitioner services followed by computerisation of doctors, dentists, etc... with the object of networking the whole health service by the year 2000. This report looks at the planning and results so far.

[198]   McCurry M: Microcomputers in General Practice - has there been any progress? Current Perspectives in HC: 65-73, BJHC, 1985.

E

An evaluation of the DTI initiative in 1982 to provide up to 150 practices with microcomputer systems. Although the uptake of computers has been slow the scheme has promoted awareness among GPs of the impact computers can have.

[199]   McDonald CJ et al: Reminders to physicians from an introspective computer medical record. A two year randomised trial. Ann Intern Med **100**(1): 130-138, 1984.

A

This system responds to its own content according to physician-authored reminder rules. To determine the effect of the reminder messages generated by 1490 rules on physician behaviour, practitioners in a general medicine clinic were randomly assigned to study or control groups. The computer's findings are reported here.

[200]   McLachlan G, Shegog RR: Computers in the Service of Medicine. Oxford University Press, 1968.

I

Two volumes devoted to the use of computers for the improvement of patient care. The first volume states the need for a flexible approach and the danger of over-early standardisation. The second looks at the problems met in analysing these medical procedures which must be clarified if systematic use of computers is to develop to full advantage.

[201]   McWilliams A: The age of the computer. JRCGP **36** (292):   490 - 491, 1986.

I An external article which looks at the purchase and expectations of a computer in general practice.

[202] McWilliams A: Information technology in general practice. The Practitioner **231**: 1034 - 1037, 1987.

E

For the vast majority of general practitioners, computers will be information tools to be used as a routine part of daily practice. There is an urgent need for this technology to be accepted so that the deeper problems of information standards may be addressed. The paper concludes "Think information".

[203] Meldrum D: Simple Computerised Disease Register. BMJ **282**: 191-194, 1981.

A/F

Disease registers, in particular those which register all diseases and all patients seen, have presented formidable problems of collating and analysing data. But the introduction of relatively cheap computers has made it practical to have simple systems for recording and analysing information on diseases. Small computers do not have adequate memory to store all the information required for age/sex registers and a disease index. The author gets round this problem by developing a combination of a manual age/sex register and a computerised disease register.

[204] Meldrum D: Simple Computerised repeat prescription control system. BMJ **282**: 1933-1937, 1981.

D

In any practice there are patients whose condition is stable but who require continuous medication. These patients do not want to see the doctor each time they need more tablets - they just want a repeat prescription. When no face-to-face consultation takes place considerable problems in monitoring and controlling arise. Micro-computers appear to offer the opportunity to control repeat prescriptions in a better way than before. So this is what the paper investigates.

[205] Michel C et al: Validation of a Knowledge Base intended for General Practitioners to assist treatment of Diabetes: A blind study. MEDINFO 86: 122-127, North-Holland , 1986.

E

This validation of SPHINX, an expert system, established the level of advice given by the system measured against that of two experts. The theories which oppose each other are reviewed by the experts in a blind study: hence it is possible to refine the experts' opinion on the quality of advice of SPHINX, and also to study the experts' assessments of their own attitudes. In a second part a sensitivity study on the interpretation by the system of laboratory data is presented.

[206] Miller RA et al: INTERNIST-1 an experimental computer-based diagnostic consultant for general internal medicine. N.EngJMed **307**: 468-476, 1982.

C

This experimental computer program is capable of making complex and multiple diagnoses in internal medicine. It differs from most other programs in the generality of its approach and the size and diversity of its knowledge base. This is a comprehensive report on the system and its capabilities.

[207]   Miller RA et al: An experimental computer based diagnostic consultant for general internal medicine. N Eng J Med. **307:** 468 -478, 1982.

C A look at INTERNIST-1, an experimental computer program capable of making multiple and complex diagnosis in the generality of its approach and the size and diversity of its knowledge base. The program has been systematically evaluated in terms of capabilities and performance.

[208]   Mohr J et al: Text Processing Systems for the doctors office. MIE 82: 262-271, Springer-Verlag , 1982.

H

A survey shows that text processing can result in economic gains and improvement of office organisation in approximately 10% of physicians' practices. One equally important motive for applying text processing is analysis of office structure and function. This means that primitive text processing techniques do not suffice. An outline for the functions of a text processing system suitable for physicians' offices is given.

[209]   Neal LR: The provision of data processing facilities for medical practitioners. MIE 78: 109-116, Springer-Verlag , 1978.

E

The present gap between the computer and the doctor who wishes to use its power needs closing by both sides - by the computing profession in providing better, easier techniques for the non expert user, and by the medical profession in accepting that education about the use of computers is an essential part of every practitioner's training.

[210]   Nicholson WH, Canning B: The benefits of a patient administration system. Current Perspectives in HC: 165-169, BJHC, 1987.

H

The paper looks at how patient administration systems (PAS) contribute to getting the NHS information act together, and especially to examine the benefits which are being realised by the extensive investment of the NHS in PAS.

[211]   Nilsson S et al: A computer in the physician's consultancy. MEDINFO 83: 1185-1186, North-Holland , 1983.

C/E

Drug prescribing is selected as an introductory project for the physician's terminal system. Computerised prescribing requires a fast and easy procedure combined with a maximum of security. Another consideration of crucial importance is to make the equipment discrete enough not to disturb the doctor-patient relationship.

[212]   Ockenden J, Bodenhamp: Focus on Medical Computer Development. OUP, 1970.

I

This is a review by a firm of consultants specialising in computer and system fields of the present position of computers in medicine in Scotland. It is a general look at the field which covers most of the topics expected in this area.

[213]　Palmer P: Computing in General Practice. Scicon Consultancy International, 1980.

E

The report looks at the current trends and uses of computing in general practice and has prepared a set of guidelines and recommendations for GPs on the way computerisation may proceed in the future. It is aimed at GPs who have not yet decided to implement a computerised system and it achieves a balance between the necessary technicality of computing and the need to be understandable to the majority of GPs.

[214]　Palombi L et al. A new system on a community oriented data base for the prevention of cardiovascular diseases in young people. MIE 87: 183-187, EDI Press, Rome, 1987.

F

A community oriented data base has been established, specifically created for prevention of cardiovascular diseases in young people. The paper looks at the need for such a system, analyses the problems and issues concerned, and looks to the future.

[215]　Pantin CFA, Merrett TG: Allergy screening using a micro-computer. BMJ **285**: 483-487.

F

A practitioner who refers a blood sample, and a questionnaire completed by the patient, to a centre where both can be analysed, will obtain enough practical information to decided whether to treat or refer the patient to a specialist. The microcomputer is therefore potentially of great value in any preliminary allergy investigation.

[216]　Payne JR, Hill DW (eds): Real Time Computing in Patient Management. Peter Peregrines, 1975.

H/I

Proceedings of a symposium set-up to exchange information about practical day to day problems in computer use and the role of computers in patient care in an attempt to predict the future pattern of computer applications both in practice and research.

[217]　Payne LC, Brown PT: An introduction to medical automation, Pitman Medical, London, 1975.

I

An exposition of the basis of automation and computerisation with particular reference to their application in an health care environment. The book stresses that everyone can understand computers and the principles involved and further, that all who seek to practice modern health care should do so.

[218]　Pelosi AJ, Lewis G: The computer will see you now. BMJ **299**: 138-139, 1989.

C

Research and clinical uses of computerised assessments must be distinguished.

[219]   Petrie JC et al: Computer-assisted shared-care in hypertension. BMJ **290:** 1960-1962, 1985.

G

A computer assisted shared-care scheme for the long term management and follow-up of hypertensive patients has been developed. The scheme aims at facilitating the exchange of clinically important information between doctors, and at achieving target levels of blood-pressure with treatment in patients at highest risk of cardiovascular events.

[220]   Peumans W: Medical Computer Applications in Daily Practice by an Independent Group of Belgian Physicians. MEDINFO 74: 85-87, Almqvist & Wiksell, 1974.

E

An independent group of physicians set up an organisation to promote computer applications in daily practice. This (Belgian) experience is that the introduction of computer applications can be done if the input is not complicated and no supplementary costs are charged to the patient.

[221]   Polter AR: Computers in general practice: the patient's voice. JRCGP **31**: 683-685, 1981.

B/E

Analysis of answers to a questionnaire on the use of computers in general practice. It highlights some of the patient's apprehension on computers and confidentiality.

[222]   Preece J: Are the GP system suppliers prepared? Practice Computing. 13 - 15, November 1989.

E System suppliers will be under increasing pressure to update their software in order to meet the demands initiated by the new GP contract and audit. A report on developments in this field.

[223]   Preece J: The use of computers in general practice. Churchill Livingstone, London, 1983.

E

Assuming no prior knowledge of computers this book provides a sound understanding of their application to general practice. The book describes the roles, uses, and benefits of computers in general practice and covers the principles upon which they operate and the methods by which they may be introduced successfully into the practice setting.

[224]   Preece JF, Hearson JR: The synopsis record card: a stepping stone to the computer. JRCGP **36**: 564-566, 1986.

A

A synopsis record card has been developed for use in general practice to provide ready reference to the important facts of the patients record. When available these cards are used in 50% of consultations. These are seen as an intermediary step in computerisation.

[225] Preece JF et al: Writing all prescriptions by computer. JRCGP **34:** 655-657, 1984.

D

By using a desktop computer to check and write all prescriptions it is possible for the general practitioner to build up a medication database which has the capacity to record response to treatment and to supply information which can be reported to a remote central drug authority on a regular basis.

[226] Pringle M: Using computers in general practice research. Practitioner **230:** 635 - 9, 1986.

E A computer is not indispensable for the general practice researcher and is no substitute for creativity. However, a computer can greatly aid the process of research by identifying patients allowing the rapid and accurate statistical analysis and being invaluable as a word processor for protocols and articles.

[227] Pringle M: Greeks bearing gifts. BMJ **295:** 738 - 9, 1987.

E An editorial comment concerning the offer of a free computer system by two companies namely AAH Medical and VAMP Health and the benefits this could bring.

[228] Pringle M: Using Computers to take patient histories. BMJ **297:** 697, 1988.

C

Information on the indications, efficacy, and possibilities of computerised patient history systems.

[229] Pringle M et al: TIMER: a new objective measure of consultation content and its application to computer assisted consultations. BMJ **293:** 20-22, 1986.

C

TIMER is a reliable and practical tool for researching the consultation, and though it has shown validity in detecting differences between consultations that use a computer and those that do not, further applications are required to establish its full value.

[230] Pringle M et al: Topic analysis: an objective measure of the consultation and its application to computer assisted consultations. BMJ **290:** 1789-1791, 1988.

C

Video tape recordings of doctors' consultations, with and without a computer present, were used to classify and compare items discussed during consultation. The results are within this report.

[231] Pringle M et al: Computers in the surgery - the patient's view. BMJ **288:** 289-291, 1984.

E

A postal survey confirmed that an appreciable minority of patients are opposed to computers being used by their doctors. The questionnaire was well designed to identify their opposition more specifically. The various grounds for opposition are aired in this article.

[232]   Pringle M et al: Computerisation: the choice. BMJ **284**: 165-168, 1982.

E

A description of the computerisation of a three partner practice where a computer handled a range of problems from repeat prescriptions to taxing salaries (PAYE) and practice accounting systems. The article describes six stages which are felt to reflect the course that many practices will travel if they decide to install a computer.

[233]   Pritchard P: The information avalanche: can the GP survive. Practitioner **229**: 877-881, 1985.

C/E

Computerised decision aids would be valuable for general practice but their development has been slow because of complexity and expense. Cheap and powerful hardware and software will soon be available, so the prospect is rapidly changing. But will general practitioners accept this new tool or suffer an increasing information overload?

[234]   Pynsent PB, Fairback JC: Computer interview for patients with back pain. J. Biomed Eng II(1): 25-29, 1989.

C

The system uses a light pen for the patient - computer interface. The questionnaire consists of over 200 multiple and single choice questions. Graphic presentations are used to identify pain patterns. The procedure has been well accepted by patients and is in routine clinical use in several hospitals.

[235]   Quaak MJ: Comparison of data gathered with the help of an automated questionnaire and medical history data out of the medical record. MIE 85: 90-97, Springer-Verlag, 1985.

C

In an outpatient clinic patients themselves answered an automated questionnaire. Thereafter an extensive medical history was taken by a medical student. Similarities and differences of the data are presented and discussed.

[236]   Quaak MJ, Van der Voort PJ: Design of and experience with an automated questionnaire for medical history taking. MIE 84: 140-145, Springer-Verlag, 1984.

C

A tool has been developed which enables a physician to compose his own questionnaire which should help answer the following questions: which possibilities are there for the use of computers in medical history taking; Is it possible to support the initial patient-doctor contact with computers; which procedures should be followed to obtain reliable data?

[237]   Quaak MJ et al: Comparisons between written and computerised patient histories. BMJ **295**: 184-186, 1987.

C

The results of this study suggest that computerised history taking is suitable for certain patients in addition to, and not as a substitute for, the oral interview with a doctor.

[238]   Rafanelli M et al: An integrated system for the general practitioner choice management. MIE 84: 552-557, Springer-Verlag, 1984.

G

An operative pattern for a management system within the Italian Health Information System using the General Register Files to simplify the choice of the General Practitioners to the user is described. After a short report about the H.I.S. organisation, the authors describe the abstract model of the system, the information flow between the system nodes and the procedures activated by particular events.

[239]   Roschetti R: Prescription Monitoring System and Evaluation of Primary Care. MIE 87: 225-229, EDI Press, Rome, 1987.

D

The principle characteristics of this system are that it is portable; it can easily be transferred from one region to another. It is based in fact on generalised software and can be used for different systems of elaboration.

[240]   Rawlins D: Development of a family linkage program. Current Perspectives in HC: 31, BJHC, 1989.

A/C

This paper describes the development of a program to link the computer-held summaries of patients' cards with those of other members of their family in general practice. The program is a valuable tool that should become widely available to assist in early diagnosis and in preventative medicine.

[241]   Rawson N, Inman W: Progress of a National Scheme for prescription-event monitoring in General Practice. MEDINFO 83: 141-144, North-Holland, 1983.

D

Prescription-event monitoring (PEM) is an inexpensive technique for monitoring the effects of drugs in large numbers of patients in general practice. PEM can be used as a method for both generating and testing hypotheses about drug safety and efficacy. Some preliminary results of the first two experiments of PEM are reported.

[242]   RCGP: Choosing a computer system. RCGP Members Reference Book, 1985.

E

A methodical approach is given by a marketing director of Vamp Health for selecting a computer system for use in a general practice. The article includes a checklist to be used during the selection process.

[243]   RCGP: Advice to members considering the current "no cost" computer systems. RCGP Publication, 1987.

E

For any practice considering the "no cost" computer schemes the college advises that each practice should examine the proposals carefully and reach its own conclusion in the light of the issues set out in this paper. Careful consideration should be given to any contract needing to be signed and benefits to the practice must be weighed against the potential costs and concerns of the wider profession as a whole.

[244] RCGP (Info Resources Centre): Computerising your practice. RCGP Publication, 1986.

E

An information pack available from the RCGP which intends to provide only a basic introduction to the subject. It provides a number of guidelines and also references to literature available on the subject as well as lists of contact telephone numbers to more experienced people in this field.

[245] RCGP: Occasional Paper 13: Computers in Primary Care. Report of the Computer Working Party. RCGP Publication, 1980.
E/I

The paper considers the desirability and feasibility of computer use in general practice. The current situation is reviewed and future developments considered with particular attention to micro-computers. The paper discusses a computerised general practice system and considers political and economic problems.

[246] Read JD: Global Prevention in primary care - the GP's role. Current Perspectives in HC: 49, BJHC, 1986.

F

The microcomputer has given medicine the tool which enables the profession to offer everyone anticipatory or preventative care of quality, quantity, and consistency. This global care should be offered from primary care - centred around GPs. In fact this will depend on how GPs and primary care respond to this challenge - the paper looks at this.

[247] Rector AL et al: A human computer interface for doctors. Current Perspectives in HC: 213-221, BJHC, 1988.

E

Improved interfaces for doctors and patients are one of the keys to exploiting advanced information for medicine. Systems must be easier and quicker to use and more directly useful before they will be widely adopted during consultations. Improved interfaces are essential to widespread acceptability of information and decision support systems.

[248] Rector AL et al: A survey of developments in medical records and information systems in the UK. MIE 78: 91-100, Springer-Verlag, 1978.
A

A large portion of this work involved studying computer-assisted medical record systems of a variety of types, although the survey extended much wider and included both manual and semi-automated methods of data recording and analysis. The results of the survey are summarised here.

[249]   Rector Al, Sheldon MG: Privacy, data decay and the long term medical record. MIE 82: 686-691, Springer-Verlag, 1982.

A/B

The medical significance of certain information in the medical record declines much more rapidly than does its potential to do harm. The protocols for accessing of and transfer of information in an automated information system should therefore be governed in part by the time since it was collected. In setting up these protocols, the potential value of the information should always be weighed against the harm it might do.

[250]   Reed RC: Transferring documents from one system to another. Comput Nurs 7(2): 58-60, 1989.

A

This article describes the technical and practical problems and advantages of transferring documents from one computer operating system to another. Those who are required to use different systems will find this information useful. The article provides general guidelines and suggests trouble-shooting procedures.

[251]   Reekie D et al: Handling information in general practice - using feature cards with computers. JRCGP 25: 369-372, 1975.

A

A two-tier system of handling information has been developed for use in general practice. Punched feature cards with the conventional patients' record cards are used for the handling of primary data in the doctor's surgery. At the same time the cards provide an input to the computer. This is especially useful when information has to be collated centrally, for more advanced statistical analysis and where multiple searches of individual feature cards are required.

[252]   Reekie D, Horden K et al: New approaches to info handling in general. BMJ 2: 162 - 166, 1974.

A

This paper describes the use of punched feature cards in a general practice for 18 months. Its advantages are the low cost, speed of information retrieval, visible statistics, computer compatibility, accuracy, confidentiality, flexibility, and simplicity of setting up and collection of information. The system encourages the doctor to ask questions about his practice and could readily be adopted in other practices.

[253]   Regester WD: The Physician's office system - How to maximise its use. MIE 84: 526-530, Springer-Verlag, 1984.

E

The paper's approach is to discuss those areas germane to getting most out of a turnkey system but are seldom discussed in literature. All systems have the financial components which usually constitute the body of a paper, but these are largely ignored but the potential buyer is presented with a guide which will spell out the differences between satisfaction and disaster.

[254]   Reggia J: Computer Assisted Medical Decision Making. Springer-Verlag, 1985.

C

The book presents a series of articles that accurately reflect the achievements of computer aided decision making in medicine and evaluates critically these methods in clinical practice. The book also glimpses at the future direction the field may be taking. The book examines the various of approaches to building computer-aided decision support systems.

[255]   Reggia JA, Tuhrim S (eds): Computer-assisted Decision Making. Springer-Verlag, 1985.

C

A comprehensive survey designed to review the research that has enabled computer technology to impart to clinical medicine, and in particular medical decision-making. The book starts with a general review and then goes into various approaches and models used in medical decision-making and then concludes with a section on related issues.

[256]   Reichertz P, Schwarz B: Computers in the Doctor's Office: System Design, Physicians Motivation & Reaction. MEDINFO 80: 886-890, North-Holland, 1980.

E

The impact and efficiency of a dedicated computer system was tested under real-life conditions in six offices of private physicians. System analytical studies about time and performance, frequency and cost analysis were supplemented by motivational and benefit analysis. This paper reports on the field test mentioned.

[257]   Reichertz PL: Computer-Aided Medical Practice oriented towards diagnosis. MEDINFO 77: 191-197, North-Holland, 1977.

C

A review of the history of computers in medical diagnosis and a description of the problems and approaches of computer aided diagnosis.

[258]   Reichertz PL et al: Results of a field test of computers for the private practice. MIE 79: 283-294, Springer-Verlag, 1979.

E

Installation of computers in offices of private physicians were evaluated. The study comprised of detailed analyses of the functional characteristics of each office before, during and after the computer installation.

[259]   Renieri A: An information system for primary care (SIMB) as a link between local and national information systems. MIE 87: 613-620, EDI Press, Rome, 1987.

G

This research project is based on a) modularity of the system; b) decentralisation of processing capacities and information; c) availability to accept other nodes relating to further health services. The experiment is aimed at operative and managerial roles of each single health service.

[260]   Reynolds MT, Richards CW: Audit of computerised recall scheme for cervical cytology. BMJ **284**: 1375-1376, 1982.

F

The Avon area health authority has been operating a computer system for cervical cytology since 1977. As practices and health authorities are forced to do the same with the closure of the national network for recall in Southport in 1982, this article assesses the accuracy of the Avon Scheme in relation to one
general practice, and compares the recall system with one based on an age/sex register compiled by the FPC.

[261]   Richards B et al: A knowledge-based system for giving expert advice to the patient in all matters relating to conception, pregnancy and childbirth. MEDINFO 89: 1183, North-Holland, 1989.

F

Present pressures on medical staff in both hospitals and GPs' surgeries mean patients (male and female) are finding themselves unable to relax and seek information or advice from clinical staff. This situation can be remedied to some extent by the provision of an informative computer system. The system will provide information, give personalised expert advice, and even test the patient's knowledge and understanding via a medical quiz. The results of using it in the surgery are proving to be quite informative.

[262]   Ridderkhoff J: Research into decision making strategies used in general practice. MIE 82: 272-279, Springer-Verlag, 1982.

C

Decision strategies can be clustered into two main directions: inductive and deductive. The characteristics of the former exist in the early generation of hypotheses and the attachment of the estimation of chances to the argumentation-steps. The latter is a process of sequential logical steps with prior probabilities attached to a limited number of hypotheses. A research protocol, according to which about 50 family physicians will be interviewed, is described.

[263]   Ridderkhoff J: Diagnostic Decision Support System. MIE 87: 242, EDI Press, Rome, 1987.

C

To be successful a support system must be as closely related to the user in his daily practice. This paper discusses some important concepts of diagnostic decision support systems related to daily clinical practice.

[264]   Rigby MJ: The National Child Health System In Practice. Current Perspectives in HC: 107-113, BJHC, 1987.

F/G

The majority of general practitioners and community health care staff are already using the National Child Health System very effectively without knowing it. All children can have their preventive health care scheduled and their health status and special requirements summarised on a system which has been tested and proven at every stage. This paper looks at the success of this system and looks at what it implies for the future.

[265]   Ritchie LD: Computers in Primary Care (Practicalities and Prospectus). Heinemann, London, 1984.

E/I

This book explores the case for, and the implications of, using computers in primary health care. A particular concern is the introduction of computer assisted record systems in primary care. Also covered are suggestions on purchasing a microcomputer for practices and security of files.

[266]   Roberts D: Dispensing with computers: not an easy task. Practice Computing. 10-12, November 1989.

D

The dispensing doctor will need to provide an efficient and economic service. The chairman of the Dispensary Doctor's Association, outlines the requirements of an effective system.

[267]   Robinson ND: General practice - a technological future. The Practitioner **230**: 867, 1986.

I

Primary care computer systems are constantly being improved and the falling costs of memory and computing power should make them more widely available and more widely used. 'Expert Systems', the linking of general practice with hospital computers, drug and medical information, databases and the uses of optical discs in medical education are discussed.

[268]   Roland M et al: Evaluation of a computer assisted repeat prescribing program in general practice. BMJ **291**: 456-458, 1985.

C

After introducing a computer-assisted repeat prescribing programme into a practice, improvements were made in several aspects of practice organisation. Time was saved by doctors and receptionists, prescriptions were produced more rapidly; drug information was improved, queries from chemists about prescriptions were reduced. The costs of the system were estimated in terms of computer operator time. Computerising prescribing data provides a source of data that may be used to enable doctors to audit their own prescribing.

[269]   Ronen I, Avitzour M: Computerisation of a Community Programme in Primary Health Care. MIE 87: 231-235, EDI Press, Rome, 1987.

F

A successful computerised programme for control and prevention of cardiovascular disease has been altered resulting in an improved database, with more complete coverage and greater accuracy. Ongoing surveillance at individual and community levels ensures activities are carried out according to protocol. Changes in the individual's treatment and in the protocol itself often result from computer feedback. Evaluation is immediately obtainable as often as required.

[270]   Rothenberg LA, Aluise JJ: Implementing an automated financial management system for medical practices. J Fam Pract **18**(5): 785-790, 1984.

H

The increase in availability, affordability, and sophistication of computer technology over the past few years has prompted the development of numerous high quality software packages for management of medical advice. To ensure a successful purchase of a system, physicians and office managers must become knowledgeable about computers and their acceptability to medical practice and then devise a strategy for the purchase of a system.

[271]   Ryan MP: A national system for primary care computing. MEDINFO 89: 697-699, North-Holland, 1989.

E/I

The General Practice Administration System Scotland has been available, free, to GPs since 1984, as is its maintenance and upgrading. However GPs have to provide hardware and consumables. A look at this system and its functions and how it provides the need for accurate and comprehensive data concerning primary care.

[272]   Salaman R et al: Telematics & general practice: An experiment of a Drug Data Bank. MEDINFO 86: 246-248, North-Holland, 1986.

C/E

Development of videotext offers important opportunities to general practitioners. It offers connection to computers and thereby grants access to knowledge and thus improves decision making. This paper reports on an experiment involving around 100 GPs connected to a drug data bank by videotext.

[273]   Salkind MR: Implementing a system in general practice. BMJ **287**: 199-201, 1983.

E

If you say to yourself "Why should I buy a computer?" and "Do I really need one?", then this article will try to answer your questions.

[274]   Salkind MR: General Practice: Hardware & Software. BMJ **287**: 106-109, 1983.

E

A look at how a practice organised itself for computerisation and some of the problems due to the unreliability of hardware and software.

[275]   Saul PD: Accessing remote data bases using micro computers. JRCGP **35**: 384-386, 1985.

A/E

GPs' access to remote data bases using micro-computers is increasing, making even the most obscure information readily available. Some of the systems available to GPs in the UK are described and the methods of access are outlined. General Practitioners should be aware of the advances in technology; data bases are increasing in size, the cost of access is falling and their use is becoming easier.

[276]   Saunderson H: Potential benefits for patient care for computing. Community Medicine. **9** (3): 238 - 246, 1987.

E

This paper covers the potential areas of benefit, reviews the most relevant evidence and offers a view on the most effective strategy for clinical computing development in the immediate future. The studies deal with primary and secondary care. However, a recent review of new technology in general practice covers the former area in some detail.

[277] Scadding JG: Diagnosis: the clinician and the computer. Lancet **2**: 877-881, 1967.

C

The interest of computers to clinical diagnosis has directed attention to the diagnostic process itself. Analysis of this process, in such a way that at least a major part of it can be performed by mathematical technique, is an essential preliminary to the use of a computer. A look at the diagnostic process and how computers can be applied to that process is the main topic of this paper.

[278] Scicon: Computers for General Practice: Conclusions of a feasibility study by Scicon Consultancy International. BMJ **2**: 884, 1980.

E

This is a summary of the feasibility study by Scicon Consultancy to determine the present and future requirements of computers for general practice. The conclusions and main recommendations are outlined here.

[279] Sheldon MG: The doctor, the patient and the computer. The Practitioner, **228**: 1121-1142, December, 1984.

E/I

There is a need for doctors to be involved in developing computer systems if they are to stay in the pivotal position in primary health care. At the heart of the general practitioner's computer will be an 'active medical record' which will reduce the burden of record keeping and provide a means of checking the doctor's actions.

[280] Sheldon MG: Using a micro-computer for doing monitoring in general practice. MIE 82: 380-386, Springer-Verlag, 1982.

F

A micro computer system was installed in a busy health centre serving 12,000 patients. Problems arose with the choice of computer hardware and operating system, methods of data
collection, entry and verification, file structure and production of output. An encounter form was designed to collect information. These problems are discussed and some of the solutions used are described.

[281] Sheldon MG: Satisfying the information needs of the general practitioner for improved patient care. MIE 78: 117-120, Springer-Verlag, 1978.

E

The GP requires a constant flow of information from various sources in order to keep himself up-to-date, to provide his patients with better advice and therapy, and to refer them to other agencies when indicated. This paper looks at ways of attaining such goals.

278

[282]   Sheldon MG: Computers in General Practice: a personal view.
         JRCGP **34**: 647-648, 1984.

E

Is the computer a devilish invention, to be avoided at all costs, or is it God's gift to general practice? - A personal opinion.

[283]   Sheldon MG: Giving patients a copy of their computer medical
         record. JRCGP **32**: 80-86, 1982.

A

A study of the views of both GPs and patients on the usefulness and acceptability of medical records. Some of the benefits and difficulties of using a computer to store medical records and of giving patients a copy of the medical summary are discussed.

[284]   Sheldon M, Stoddard N: Trends in General Practice Computing.
         RCGP, 1985.

I

A collection of articles written by GPs with experience of computers in their practices. Covers all the important areas of computing in general practice, personal views, and looks into the future.

[285]   Shepherd SG: Comprehensive Preventative Medicine in General
         Practice: a new role for the micro-computer. Current Perspectives in
         HC: 53-64, BJHC,1989.

F

Preventative medicine and follow up treatment are becoming ever more important in primary care. A number of screening measures which fulfil all the strictest criterion, save lives and are cost effective are described. Prevention can even save time. The case for prevention has never been stronger. How and where do micro-computers fit in?

[286]   Shortliffe E, Claney W: Readings in Medical Artificial Intelligence: the
         first decade. Addison-Wesley, 1984.

I

An excellent encapsulation of past A.I. research in medicine, comprising reprints of the seminal articles with perceptive chapters, introductions, and epilogues.

[287]   Simon P, Naszlady A: Memory Card - Micro Chip - In Primary Health
         Care. MEDINFO 86: 1015-1018, North-Holland, 1986.

A

Personal computers and the appearance of memory cards open the way up for developing systems to help support the management of the medical services, the preventive-curative activities, and follow-up of patients. Economical spreading of these systems and their social acceptability are facilitated by their ability to offer a scale of different services.

[288]   Singer G, Hall G: Results of a Primary Health Care Data Base.
         Current Perspectives in HC: 48, BJHC, 1989.

A

Until recently data was relatively inaccessible in the NHS because the written records were in a manual filing system. With the introduction of computer systems into general practice this situation has changed and groups of patients can be easily identified for research purposes. The development of a data bank of anonymised patient records provides an excellent source of primary care data for a range of medical research and planning projects.

[289]   Skinner HA et al: Lifestyle assessment: applying micro computers in family pactice. BMJ **290**: 212-214, 1985.

F

Histories of alcohol, tobacco, and drug use were obtained by computer, interview, and questionnaire. Patients gave differential ratings about the method of assessment. The computer rated more interesting but also cold and impersonal; patients who completed the assessment by computer showed a significant increase in their preference for computers after the assessment. The results indicate that patient acceptance of computers may be favourably influenced by direct experience with a microcomputer.

[290]   Smith C: Computer Programme to Estimate Recurrence Risks for Multifactorial Familial Disease. BMJ **1**: 495-497, 1972.

F

A computer programme to estimate recurrence risks for multifactorial genetic disease in affected families uses parameters on population prevalence, on the inheritability of the condition, and details of the family history. Information on affected and unaffected relatives, on sex, or age effects on prevalence and on inheritability, can all be accommodated by the programme.

[291]   Soljak MA, Handford S: Early results from the Northland immunisation register. NZ Med J **100**(822): 244-246, 1987.

F

Birth information has been recorded and used to study two interventions aimed at increasing immunisation levels in an experimental group. The first involves sending to general practitioners lists of infants due for immunisation, and the second sending immunisation reminder cards to parents. Results show significant differences in immunisation levels between test group infants and comparable controls.

[292]   Somerville S, et al: MICKIE - Experiences in taking histories from patients using a microcomputer. MIE 79: 713-721, Springer-Verlag, 1979.

C

A questionnaire is presented to the patient on a computer terminal. The patient responds to questions by pressing one of the buttons marked 'yes', 'no', 'don't know', and 'don't understand'. The computer logs the response and presents the next question in the logical sequence based on previous answers. At the end of the interview the computer prints a 'summary' which is then seen by the doctor.

[293]   South J: A computer summary used as a discharge letter. JRCGP **22**: 28-32, 1972.

E

A summary of pregnancy, labour, and the puerperium has been sent routinely to the general practitioner when a mother is discharged from one of the St. Thomas Hospital Maternity Units since 1970. This obsteric summary has been produced by a computer from coded obstetric records. The report also gives the response by general practitioners.

[294]   Stevens RG, Crabbe AM: Computerised Patient Retained Records: A Working System. Current Perspectives in HC: 250-261, BJHC, 1985.

A

Increased mobility among patients and doctors and the development of health care teams places a strain on conventional patient management resources. An efficient service relies on good communication between doctors and allied health care professionals. This requires an accurate, integrated record system; a fundamental requirement which is not currently met.

[295]   Stevens R, Crabbe A: Experiences with Computer Card Medication Records in Britain. MIE 88: 180-184, Springer-Verlag, 1988.

D

These cards can be used for two-way communication between doctors and pharmacists. Records of drugs bought over the counter by the patient can be added to the card by the pharmacist. Similarly, endorsement of the card when drugs are dispensed indicates to the doctor that the patient has acutally presented the prescription.

[296]   Stimson DH et al: A problem-oriented information system for a primary care group practice. MEDINFO 77: 463-466, North-Holland, 1977.

A

A computer base information system was developed to support a primary care group practice, and is designed to provide data about patients as well as patient visits, to estimate costs of serving those with chronic illnesses, and to relate drugs prescribed, tests ordered, and procedures done for each patient, to a specific problem on the patient's problem list.

[297]   Stoddart N: The Computer in General Practice. The Practitioner **227**: 1825 - 1835, 1983.

E

Although the use of micro-computers in general practice is still at an early stage, there are already indications that the machine will be of great help to the GP. It envisages how the computer could expand from its present narrow use to the wider medical community so that a GP could, for instance, receive up-to-minute information on progress of patients in hospital.

[298]   Studin JR, Kalisman M: Computers and Medical Office Management. Clin Plast Surg **13**(3): 367-374, 1986.

H

This article outlines the possible uses of computers and software in the management of a medical office. It highlights many issues that should be considered in choosing a system.

[299] Sullivan D, Victor CR: Using computers for health education in general practice: a pilot study. Computers in Health Care Education and Training, 1988.

F

One method of increasing the preventative element of general practice is via health education and health promotion techniques. Traditional means of health education promotion is time consuming although effective. This study examines the potential of computers to provide effective health education using a technique called Health Risk Appraisal. The study assesses three different types of program and the patient attitude to each.

[300] Sweeney J et al: Benefits of an integrated community system. Current Perspectives in HC: 122-128, BJHC, 1987.

G

This paper is based on work carried out with a number of health authorities and outlines the scope of community health services, the distinctive characteristics of second-generation systems, the functions and benefits of a community patient-care system, and the additional benefits of a district patient care system.

[301] Symington et al: Shared-Care Project. Current Perspectives in HC: 19-21, BJHC, 1989.

E

Many problems in long term patient care stem from inadequate communication and lack of coordination. A shared care scheme attempts to overcome these problems and to provide good quality care for patients through an appropriate balance of specialist and general practice provision, with more cost-effective use of health care resources. The article describes a shared-care scheme for hypertension in the West of Scotland.

[302] Tanner S: Expert Systems: starting small. Practice Computing 5(9), 1987.

I

Most developments in expert systems take place in the rarefied atmosphere of the universities. But the computer's ability to analyse information and reach conclusions based on all relevant factors can be exploited much closer to home.

[303] Taylor TR et al: Doctors as Decision Makers: A computer assisted study of diagnosis as a cognitive skill. BMJ 3: 35-40, 1971.

C

When viewed as a sequence of decisions, clinical diagnosis becomes amenable to detailed investigation in terms of standard statistical concepts. Considerable variation in the rates of correct diagnosis is shown when these rates are compared in detail to five statistical measures related to the effective use of information available to the clinicians. For rapid analysis of diagnostic skill two visual methods are presented.

[304] Telling JP et al: Developing a practice formulary as a by-product of computer controlled repeat prescribing. BMJ **288**: 1730-1732, 1984.

D

An office computer is used to record and issue repeat precriptions. Monthly a printout is examined to see how many times a drug has been prescribed with the goal of limiting the practice formulary. The GPs have reduced the range of drugs prescribed by 10% and have the possibility of knowing dose ranges, actions, interactions, and side effects of all the drugs used in the practice.

[305]   Temmerman G et al: PLUSOMR - A microcomputer POMR-SYSTEM
for Primary Care. MEDINFO 83: 1173-1176, North-Holland, 1983.

A

The system allows the general practitioner to carry out medical management and to retrieve relevant clinical data. It also constitutes the basis for a number of further useful applications such as referral letters. The system is eminently suitable for the training of medical students in case recording and evaluation.

[306]   Temmerman G, Plumans W: A modular integrated medical record
for general practice. MIE 79: 261-271, Springer-Verlag, 1979.

A

Belgian physicians have gradually become aware of the help computers can give in their daily work. The project pays special attention to the feasibility of an automated medical record and to the improvement of health care induced by its use. From the created data base, statistical studies on morbidity, mortality, and practice analysis could be made possible.

[307]   Thome R: Protection and Confidentiality of Medical Data - Efficient
Data Protection through project specific combination of methods.
MEDINFO 74: 189-191, Almqvist & Wiksell, 1974.

B

Some problems with the German law concerning data security are aired and a method is described by which an appropriate and economical combination of protective measures can be determined.

[308]   Timpka T: Introducing hypertext in primary health care: a study on
the feasibility of decision support for practitioners. Comput Methods
Programs Biomed **29**(1): 1-13, 1989.

C

A study on the feasibility of the introduction of hypertext systems for communication of medical knowledge in primary care is described. Shortliffe's constraints on areas for application of decision support are evaluated.

[309]   Timpka T et al: Decision Support for General Practitioners: Design
and Implementation by Integrating Paradigms: Hypertext, Knowledge
Based Systems and Online Library. MEDINFO 86: 96-100,
North-Holland, 1986.

C

Most decision support systems (DSSs) in medicine have been developed in the hospital environment, only a few have been developed for use by GPs in primary care. The work reported in this paper has a twofold aim: (1) designing DSS for GPs in primary care, considering the social context of patient encounters, and (2) integration of three approaches; Hypertext, Knowledge Based Systems, and Online Library, since only one will not suffice for the varying needs of the GP.

[310]   Timpka T, Arborelius E: Study of the practitioner's knowledge need and use during health care consultations: Theory and Method. MEDINFO 89: 689-693, North-Holland, 1989.

C

Study of the knowledge use and needs of practitioners is an important topic in medical informatics, with relevance for educational design and organisation development, as well as in the design of Decision Support Systems. No scientific methods are, up to this date, available for the study of these issues in the consultation situation. In this paper is presented a method based on 'continental' phenomenology, focusing on the practitioner's need of 'reflection in action' and the relational basis for communication in the consultation process.

[311]   Trower C: Data for Prevention - how GPs can do it. Current Perspectives in HC: 22-28, BJHC, 1988.

F

Perhaps the only logical place for the collection and analysis of data prevention is by the primary health care team in general practice. The information can then be aggregated for health care planning or given back to the individual to encourage personal responsibility for health. The paper aims to demonstrate that not only can general practice be responsible for data prevention, but indeed, it should be.

[312]   Tsubo T: Safety and Security of Medical Information Systems. MEDINFO 80: 308-310, North-Holland, 1980.

B

A look at today's maintenance of safety and security of medical information taking into consideration the changes in information required from systems and the value of patient care.

[313]   Tsumura H et al: Patient Oriented Multidisciplinary Medical Consultation System. MEDINFO 86: 289-293, North-Holland, 1986.

C

A system, DOCTORS, has been designed to be used by both doctors and patients to answer the problem of uncertainty, by both parties, as to the area of medical speciality that applies to a given disease. The system is in use for the initial stages of diagnosis in consultations.

[314]   Turner RD et al: Computers in primary care: where next? BMJ 2: 1020-1022, 1980.

I

This paper looks at the state of computerisation and evaluates the cost-effectiveness of computerising a practice, how to select a computer, and how to evaluate it. It also addresses the problem of confidentiality.

[315]   UpJohn Fellowship Report: Simple computer facilities in general practice. JRCGP: 19: 269-281, 1970.

284

E

Literature on morbidity recording, and the use of computer facilities, is reviewed; an exercise in continuous morbidity recording with simple computer facilities is referred to, and some of the problems encountered are enumerated.

[316]   Uplekor MW et al: Sympmed I: computer program for primary health care. BMJ **297**: 841-843, 1988.

F

Sympmed I is an experimental computer program that identifies and offers treatment to outpatients whose symptoms can be effectively and safely treated. To verify the safety of such a package an evaluation was carried out which confirmed that most problems seen by first level medical staff in developing countries are simple, repetitive, and treatable at home by a paramedical worker with a few safe, essential drugs, thus avoiding unnecessary visits to a doctor.

[317]   Vallbona C et al: Use of a computerised data base to monitor the level of control of hypertension in community health centres. MEDINFO 83: 261-264, North-Holland, 1983.

F

To improve hypertension control of a low-income population in Houston, a protocol was introduced in 1975 to give physicians instructions for screening, diagnosis, step care/drug management, and compliance/follow-up monitoring. In 1979 the protocol was updated ensuring early treatment of borderline hypertensives and providing guidelines for physician-patient communications. The protocol's impact has been assessed and this paper reports on the design and results of the system.

[318]   Van Egmond J, Wieme RJ: COMPADOS: How to convince a physician to use a computerised medical record system. MIE 78: 339-349, Springer-Verlag, 1978.

A

One of the objectives of the computerised medical record system COMPADOS is to convince the individual physician of its advantages for patient care, medical research, medical education, and health care management. The project is discussed in this paper.

[319]   Vansteenland H: MEDOC: medical documents on computer. MIE 84: 558-564, Springer-Verlag, 1984.

A

MEDOC is a software package offering a fully personalised Data Management of the medical file, a complete administrative and financial control of the medical practice, book-keeping, a scientific approach to a medical databank with statistical retrieval and processing, and a personal information system for the practitioner. This paper looks at the package.

[320]   Vohloren I: Measurement of Productivity in Primary Care. MIE 85: 399-403, Springer-Verlag, 1985.

I

The aim of this paper is to present some results from a study measuring the productivity in primary curative care, and to suggest some recommendations for nationwide monitoring of primary care services.

[321]   Walker CH: "Batch" or "on-line" for child health - a review. BMJ **281**: 90-92, 1980.

I

A look at two actual systems. One is online, the other batch. The review assesses the suitability of each method with reference to important issues such as accuracy, confidentiality, security, safeguards and cost, and draws some appropriate conclusions.

[322]   Watkins GB: Computerisation of a diabetic clinic records. BMJ **281**: 1402-1403, 1980.

A

A simple system has been developed by using stationery that combines the usual handwritten records with the minimum of suitable data for punching onto a computer tape. The record may be brought up-to-date at a selected time interval. The information is mainly used for research, but does aid administration.

[323]   Weeks R: For all those about to go online...... GP: August 21, 1987.

E

Dr. Roger Weeks advises on how to go about installing a computer in your practice.

[324]   Welch J: Computerised information retrieval services in a teaching hospital. BMJ **280**: 1433-1434, 1980.

F

An increasing number of institutions provide an on-line information retrieval system for medical research and teaching staff. This is an overview of the current facilities available.

[325]   White DH: The Computer Health Check - the first 100 patients. JRCGP **34**: 661-663, 1984.

C

While waiting to see a doctor, patients used a computerised interview to answer questions about their health. An analysis of the first 100 interviews is presented. The results indicate that patients like the system and doctors find it useful.

[326]   Whitehouse CR: Preparing to introduce a computer into a Health Centre. BMJ **283**: 107-110, 1981.

E

If computers are to be introduced successfully into a medical environment, then there must be a firm commitment by the medical and office staff. Therefore, if it is necessary to alter staff attitudes or working practice, this should be asssessed beforehand. An attempt (this report) was made to assess the attitudes of staff to using a computer in one Health Centre.

[327]   Williamson JD: Data protection and the clinician: guidelines on data security. BMJ **291**: 1516-1519, 1985.

B

A look at the advent of the computer and the data protection issues that go with it, the implications, and a recommended code of practice.

[328]   Willis A: GP Computer Systems. Pulse Reviews 1987.

E

A set of reviews of GP computer systems after a 2 hour demonstration of each. The intention is to illustrate a method of assessing systems. It is important to look at the company as well as the currently available software. It suggests practices choosing a system should consider operational detail very carefully. A demonstration, it should be noted, makes an invaluable impression of the system.

[329]   Willis A, Stewart T: Computers: A Guide to Choosing and Using.
           Oxford University Press, 1989.

I

Looks at what the practitioner is trying to achieve and whether a computer would help. Takes into account considerations required before implementation. How to choose a system - what to look for, how to obtain and install the system and maintain it. Also looks at business applications and the future.

[330]   Willis J: Bringing the visiting diary up to date. BMJ **292**: 1715-1716,
           1986.

E

A method is described for the systematic assessment and review of long term dependent patients in a small practice using a personally developed computer program and assessment scale.

[331]   Young DW: A survey of decision aids for clinicians. BMJ **285**:
           1332-1335, 1982.

I

Inconsistency in applying medical knowledge is a major reason for having varying standards of medical care. Five types of aid have been introduced to help medical decision making: questionnaires, algorithms, database systems, diagnostic systems, and computer-based decision support systems. Of these, the most effective act as reminder or prompt systems to assist doctors without threatening their clinical freedom.

[332]   Anon: The impact of a micro computer on a practice immunisation
           clinic. The Practitioner **232**: 197, 1988.

A/F

Both written and computerised records have been kept on children attending a general practice immunisation clinic. The use of a computer has greatly eased the task of producing up-to-date immunisation rates to show parents in an attempt to improve immunisation uptake.

[333]   Anon: The long road to Government funding of GP systems.
           Practice Computing: 8-10, September 1989.

I

The problem of funding computers has been the main obstacle to their introduction into general practice. The article reviews strategies for dealing with the problem.

[334] Anon: The Data Protection Act: more questions than answers. Practice Computing: 11-14, September 1989.

B

Not formed with medical information in mind, the DPA raises important questions and issues for GPs. This article provides a guide through the jungle of legislation.

[335] Anon: Flying Start with a desktop network. Practice Computing: 19-20, February, 1989.

E

The partners and staff of a Derby practice saw a GP computer system that immediately gained their confidence, so they took the plunge installing six stations on one day. Their initial experience has been very positive: as described here the system has demanded little time and been easy to integrate into the practice.

[336] Anon: GP database - community resource. Practice Computing: 12-18, February 1989.

G

The free exchange of information between GPs and FPCs and health authorities has enormous advantages. A project aims to demonstrate that GPs' computers not only benefit their practices but provide information to help run local services.

[337] Anon: Linking FPC and GP Systems. Practice Computing: 7-10, February 1989.

G

The interrogation of FPC computers by GP systems in the IOS or reimbursement area is being evaluated. The system appears to be a definitive step forward.

[338] Anon: Health Screen - the only real cure is prevention. Practice Computing: 9-14, November 1988.

F

About a health screening program now in operation at a Health Centre which is striking in its simplicity, directness of approach, and cost effectiveness. Patient response - and the increasing readiness of colleagues to encourage patients to undergo the program - is proving highly encouraging.

[339] Anon: Diabetes: rapid strides in computerised control. Practice Computing: 4-8, November 1988.

F

Rapid technological advances associated with the management of diabetes are now being made. The article draws opinions from interviews with experts in the field about the emergence of the reflectance meter for enhanced diabetic control.

[340] Anon: Screen Management: a view of the future? Practice Computing: 5-9, September 1988.

C

A look at what exactly using a computer in the consulting room involves. Vamp Health provide a scenario giving a flavour of how effective it can be.

[341]   Anon: Does a computerised practice make perfect? Practice Computing: 7-11, May 1988.

E

What impact have the "free schemes" had on practices looking to computerise? How do rival systems compare? Practice Computing visits a dispensing practice which is currently addressing the complex issues involved in selecting a suitable system.

[342]   Anon: Ten Questions for the free computer suppliers. Practice Computing Autumn 1987.

E/I

The 'free schemes' are not simple: they raise a lot of issues. VAMP's and AAH Medicals chief executives answer some of the questions that have been raised.

[343]   Anon: Required reading for computer buyers. Practice Computing 1986 **4**(4): 26-27, February 1986.

E

The article says why the "Micros for GPs" is required reading for any practice contemplating installing one, and talks about the impact of change on the practice, the need to prepare for change, the effect of innovative equipment and procedures, and the problem of building up a new set of relationships.

[344]   Anon: Reaping High Rewards (from an inexpensive system). Practice Computing **4**(4): 14-17, February 1988.

E

A look at a practice where a low-cost computer is being used to great effect. In terms of service to patients, the advantages have been dramatic.

[345]   Anon: Ensuring that GPs can control confidentiality. Practice Computing: 16-17, Summer 1987.

B

Much concern is being expressed about the issue of confidentiality of data in relation to the two 'free' computer packages now on offer to GPs. Each supplier offers a different approach to confidentiality - but in the end it is the doctor who must decide.

[346]   Anon: Computerisation: A Methodical Approach. Practice Computing **4**(3): 4-7, 1985.

E

The care you put into selecting a computer and introducing it into the practice should pay dividends. This is a report from a Buckingham practice which, within a year of laying down the proper foundations, has begun to reap major benefits.

[347]   Anon: A Stand on Standards. Practice Computing **4**(2): 5-7, 1985.

I

It is argued here that standards are essential if the present diversity of practice computing systems is to evolve. While standardisation of systems is a very long way of it appears there is no lack of standards to be going on with.

[348]   Anon: A question of communication. Practice Computing April **4**(1): 8-12, 1985.

E

This article reports that computers do not work in isolation - they need to be integrated with the everyday working of the practice and often new procedures are needed so that the benefits of using computers can be realised. Also described is the way one practice handles communication between patient, doctor, and the office computer in the context of repeat prescribing.

[349]   Anon: A quite bright future. Practice Computing December 1984.

I

The paper draws on the Alvey Directorate and emphasises a practical realisation of computers and computer techniques which is both reassuring and intriguing. The author allays contemporary fears of computer use and puts the computer firmly in its place. The paper concludes with 'An Awful Warning' concerning legal liability and computer use.

[350]   Anon: Checklist for computing. Practice Computing Oct. 1984.

E

Choosing a computer system that will do the job properly is largely a matter of asking the right questions. A number of areas are identified in which computers should be assessed - and suggests the questions to ask on each area.

[351]   Anon: A Tale of Two Systems. Practice Computing April 1984.

E

You can look on a computer as an extra pair of hands to help out in the office, or you can try to take it further; we look at the experiences of two practices who are exploring some of the possibilities.

[352]   Anon: Picking and Choosing (a system for a practice). Practice Computing **3**(2): 6-8, 1984.

E

Practices are increasingly well informed about the functions a computer could perform for them, and its impact on the practice when it comes to choosing a specific system. A healthy scepticism is recommended and also offered are some assessment criteria.

[353]   Anon: Seizing the opportunity. Practice Computing **3**(1): 23-24, 1984.

A

Swooping hardware costs make it feasible to link patient history with patient records within the practice system - the problem is how to do it.

[354]   Anon: Computers in Perspective. Practice Computing **3**(1): 16-17, 1984.

I

The micros for GPs scheme has come in for a lot of criticism, however much of it is ill-informed. The article argues for a more open attitude to help dispel misconceptions, and points out a few home-truths.

[355]   Anon: How to live happily with a computer. Practice Computing 2(5): 20-22, 1983.

E

After the effort of selecting a computer system the effort should not stop. Sound maintenance and effective use of the computer system can greatly increase the chance of it benefiting the GP, the staff, and patients.

[356]   Anon: Any Questions - computer interviewing. Practice Computing 12(5): 18-19, 1983.

C

A look at the considerable scope in general practice for computer interviewing and a look at why general practitioners have been slow to consider it.

[357]   Anon: The Electronic Notebook. Practice Computing 2(4): 18-20, 1983.

C

A look at computer techniques for patient interviewing are a valuable adjunct to more conventional techniques. The article explains why.

[358]   Anon: The Next Step. Practice Computing 2(4): 11-12, 1983.

E

When buying a computer for general practice the questions to ask may be: should I buy now or wait? and what should I look for in a vendor? The article addresses these questions.

[359]   Anon: Computer Forum 1. Forum between RCGP and BCS. Practice Computing 2(3): 8-13, 1983.

I

No critique.

[360]   Anon: Past, Present and Future. (History and development of Practice Systems). Practice Computing 2(2): 24-25, 1983.

I

A brief history and development of practice systems, what they comprise of in basic form, the possibilities resulting from the basic systems, and prospects for their future.

[361]   Anon: Repeat Performer: (on repeat prescription systems). Practice Computing 2(2): 18-23, 1983.

D

Repeat prescriptions are seen as a convenience for the patient, and so, the more convenient repeat prescribing can be made with the use of computers the greater the likelihood of compliance.

[362]   Anon: Computers in Care: studying care for the chronically ill.
Practice Computing 1(6): 18-21, 1982.

E

Two practices in Sheffield are taking part in a unique exercise studying the care of the chronically sick. The article looks at the impact a computer can have on the long term management of such patients and the quality of care that such a system could bring about.

[363]   Anon: Computer Manager. Practice Computing 1(5): 22-23, 1982.

H

A discussion about the ways a computer can help in long term patient management. A look at patient attitudes, their apparent lack of concern, and the possible impact computers could have.

[364]   Anon: Where do we go from here? the next step for computing in general practice. Practice Computing 1(5): 19-21, 1982.

I

A look at the next step for computing in general practice and the developments and future to look forward to.

[365]   Anon: Counting Costs - how much will a computer cost you?
Practice Computing 1(4): 6-8, 1982.

E

How do you calculate the real cost of ownership of a computer? A GP computer system supplier explains how to work out costs.

[366]   Anon: High tech response to a new NHS hits obstacles.
Medeconomics: July 1989.

I

The requirements of the NHS review demand that GPs be equipped with standardised systems. But lack of information means that the necessary software is not yet on hand.

[367]   Anon: The future of GP computing is taking shape now.
Medeconomics: May 1989.

I

As technology develops, it is likely that more information will only be available to GPs from computers. Having one on every desk will therefore become a necessity.

[368]   Anon: Computer suppliers vie for GPs custom. Medeconomics:
March 1989.

I

The GP micro market is thriving as 'giveaway' schemes compete with traditional suppliers. The result will benefit all GPs who are, or who plan to be, computerised.

[369]   Anon: Practice buys into the computer age. Medeconomics:
February 1989.

E

Over a year the journal is to follow the fortunes of a practice computerisation project. This, the first part of the series, describes how the practice fared on day one. A step by step guide is provided for GPs wishing to do the same.

[370]   Anon: Value for money is more than a big name. Medeconomics: January 1989.

E

Buying a household name may be reassuring to the novice but it is a needlessly costly exercise - the title says it all.

[371]   Anon: Get advice on making the most of a GP computer. Medeconomics: January 1988.

E

A number of nationwide schemes are now offering advice to GPs taking their first steps in practice computing.

372]Anon: Count costs to maintain your computer. Medeconomics: February 1987.

E

The article advises a long, hard look at the terms of your maintenance contract before you commit yourself to investing in a computer for your practice.

[373]   Anon: Computers in Practice: 3 part series. Pulse April 1988.

E

This series looks at what a computer can do for a practice, advises GPs on how to choose equipment and looks at computers and the Data Protection Act. The series concludes with reports from GPs already using computers and looks at the future.

[374]   Anon: Evaluating medical computer systems. N.Z. Family Physician: Spring 1988.

E

The importance of adequate software and company support is stressed. Together with personal commitment, these will ensure a successful installation. Important aspects of the contract are described and a 'score sheet' is provided as a basis for evaluating different schemes.

[375]   Anon: Introducing expert systems to medical students using ESTA, Expert System Teaching Aid. Medical Education 22: 99-103, 1988.

I

ESTA is a computer model of an expert system, developed to make the best use of time allocated to medical students. The nature of the interaction with ESTA is described and their reactions to the expert systems in medicine are described. A discussion of these reactions draws some conclusions about teaching expert systems and computers on medical courses.

[376]   Anon: Computerisation in primary health care. The Medical Annual: 1986.

I

Over the last few years the NHS recognised the need for a population register to show who customers are, where they move to and where they come from. Since FPC's are the best sources of such data there is now the urgent need to computerise them. The paper describes the current state of FPC computing and the uses to which the FPC register could be put.

[377]   Anon: Computers in General Practice. Maternal and Child Health: 107, April 1989.

E

The number of general practices turning to computers is forever increasing. Computers contribute to effective preventive care within the community when used by the family doctor. In a practice the computer should cope with cervical smear recalls, immunisations, and all repeat prescriptions. The uses, advantages, and disadvantages of computers in general practice are discussed.

[378]   Anon: Why doctors don't use computers: some empirical findings. J. Royal Society of Medicine **79**: 1986.

I

Attitudes of students and practising physicians were taken and the following deduced: the groups are uncertain as to the possible effects on their traditional role and practice organisation. However they recognise computer potential to improve patient care, but are concerned about increases in government and hospital control and also privacy, legal, and ethical problems.

[379]   Anon: Computerising FPC registers. JRCGP **32**: 67, 1982.

G

The DHSS has recommended computerisation of registration work undertaken by FPCs. Does this signal the end of these friendly and efficient officers and staff at the local FPC and the beginning of a cold, uncommunicative computer.

[380]   Anon: Computers in Primary Care. JRCGP **30**: 387-388, 1980.

I

Compatible computer systems could, and should, be in widespread use in general practice in five years time, and be adopted by virtually all practices in ten years.

[381]   Anon: Evaluating Feasibility and Selection of Computers in Family Medicine. Journal of Family Practice **19**(1): 86-92, 1984.

E

The article addresses many of the issues, concerns, and approaches that the family physician should take when evaluating potential applications and purchase of a computer for a practice.

[382]   Anon: A study of patients' attitudes to computer interrogation. Int. J. Man-Machine Studies **9**: 69-86.

C

A report on a study which was carried out to assess patients' reactions to computer interrogation.

[383]   Anon: GP Contract 1990 Survival Guide. GP: Nov/Dec. 1989.

E

A step by step guide to installing computers in general practice. It covers all aspects of selection and installation, including training of practice-staff effectively, and adopting office routine. Also suggestions are made on how to cope with the changes that are frequently imposed on general practice.

[384]   Anon: Taking the trauma out of a new practice computer. Financial
          Pulse **3**(21), 1988.

E

Some doctors shy away from computers as the great unknown but this report shows that they can be mastered simply and also says that it is particularly important to find a system the staff can use.

[385]   Anon: Learning how to manage computerised accounts. Financial
          Pulse: 23 April 1988.

H

A report on how one general practitioner taught himself how to program his computer and how this helped improve his practice management.

[386]   Anon: Are you making the most of your practice computer?
          Financial Pulse **3**(6): 26 March, 1988.

E

Recognition that many of the difficulties encountered with practice computers are common to many GPs led the journal to visit a GP with the Chairman of the BCS Primary Health Care Specialist Group to highlight some of the problems GPs can face.

[387]   Anon: Two-year experience in problem oriented records of primary
          health care. MEDINFO 77: 479-480, North-Holland, 1977.

A

The results of a pilot project dealing with problem-oriented medical records are presented and discussed. This project took place in seven primary health care regions over a 2 year period.

[388]   Anon: Free GP systems become comparable. BJHC **4** (5): 7, 1987.

E

A short comparison of the two free schemes for GP computer systems as put forward by AHH Medical and VAMP in terms of functionality, costs, and obligations.

[389]   Anon: Computers in medicine: searching for the rainbow and the
          crock of gold. BMJ **284**: 1859-1860, 1982.

I

A rather critical look at computers in medicine and general practice from an author who claims the recent conference organised by the BMA and IEE, as a contribution to IT Year, spent too much time dreaming of the future and not enough concentrating on the brutal present.

[390]   Anon: A computer in every surgery? BMJ **280**: 1556, 1980.

E

A working party of the RCGP produced a report 'Computers in Primary Care' which enthusiastically denies misplaced apprehension of computer use and pushes for widespread use of computers in general practice. This paper takes a look at the report.

[391]   Anon: Confidentiality, records, and computers. BMJ **1**: 698-699, 1979.

B

The widening use of computers has focused the issue of confidentiality more sharply, as people become more concerned about what information is kept about them, how secure it is and what it is used for. Even with the introduction of legislation the problem is not yet solved.

[392]   Anon: Computers and Confidentiality. BMJ **2**: 1663, 1978.

B

After the publication of the report by Sir Norman Lindop's expert committee much doubt about confidentiality and the handling of the problem still exists.

[393]   Anon: Computers and Privacy. BMJ **1**: 178-179, 1976.

B

An article which discusses the current state of affairs on the titled topic, and addresses the questions and possible solutions concerned with confidentiality.

[394]   Anon: Computers and Confidentiality in Medicine. (Conference Report from 27th WM Assy.). BMJ **4**: 290-292, 1973.

B

A paper covering most of the aspects related to confidentiality and computers in medicine. The paper draws from many other papers presented at the conference covering the legal position, conflict of interest, misunderstanding, preservation of confidentiality, and anonimity in research.

[395]   Anon: Expert Systems. BJHC: 40, January 1986.

I

Expert Systems allow computers to 'think' for themselves. This article outlines the theory behind them and their application to medicine to date.

[396]   Anon: Scottish Health Computing. BJHC: January 1986.

I

An outline of the development to date of computing in the NHS in Scotland and plans for the future.

[397]   Anon: IT for GPs. BJHC: 26-35, July 1988.

G

Recent years have seen considerable growth in the number of computer systems installed in general practices and in departmental activity in GP computing. The article describes the role of the DHSS in GP computing.

[398]   Anon: A computer managed screening programme for the pre-symptomatic detection of cervical neoplasia. Current Perspectives in HC: 207-218, BJHC, 1984.

F

Primary prevention of cervical cancer remains problematic since the precise cause continues to evade elucidation. Screening, as a preventive measure is becoming an important issue. The paper looks at a computer managed technique of screening.

[399]   Anon: A computer in the pracice: Lessons learned in Sheffield. Computer Update: Autumn 1984.

E

An assessment of the pros and cons of a computer in the practice. Written by a GP, who became involved in a 3 year research project with IBM and Sheffield University to evaluate the use of computers in general practice.

[400]   Anon: Knowledge-Based decision support for general practitioners: an integrated design. Computer Methods and Programs in Biomedicine **25**: 49-60, 1987.

C

The work in this paper aims to design decision support systems (DSS) for GPs in primary care taking into consideration that primary care is the first level in a health care organisation, where the reasons for the patients' attendance are seen in a social context; and integrate three approaches - Hypertext, Knowledge-Based Systems and On Line Library - since any of these alone will not suffice for the varying needs of GPs.

[401]   Anon: How to choose a general practice computing system: comparison of commercial packages. BMJ **297**: 838-840, 1988.

E

Practitioners considering computerising their patients' records are faced with a bewildering choice of software systems. The availability of independent advice and guidance on computer systems for general practitioners varies from region to region but is generally poor. The Oxford Community Health Project has developed experience in this area of advice and describes how they obtained information on various systems and the facilities available in them.

[402]   Anon: Do personal computers make doctors less personal? BMJ **296**: 1446-1448, 1988.

C

A comparison and survey of patients views before and after a computer system was installed in their practice. Their views on a personal relationship with the doctor, duration of consultation and privacy are reported on. The study showed patients had little difficulty in accepting a computer in the consultation room. However, doctors should allay apprehension about decreases in privacy.

[403]   Anon: Combined computer generated discharge documents and surgical audit. BMJ **292**: 816-818, 1986.

A

A computerised audit system using a commercially available database programme and a word-processing programme was devised to produce discharge documents close to the time of discharge. The data were available for audit of the surgical unit's work. It was found that secretarial time was more efficiently used and general practitioners received more information about their patients earlier than before.